Computational Drug Interaction For Disease Diagnosis

Faizaan

Table of Contents

CHAPTER 1
INTRODUCTION

1.1 Fundamentals of Drug Interaction Modeling

The discovery and development of novel therapeutic agents need a thorough comprehension of how chemical compounds interact with biological systems. At the core of this endeavor lies the ability to systematically characterize and predict the relationships between drugs, their molecular targets, and the disease phenotypes they modulate. Over the last two decades, computational biology and bioinformatics have substantially advanced this field by enabling the integration of heterogeneous biological, chemical, and clinical data into predictive frameworks. Among the various conceptual pillars of computational drug discovery, three domains form the foundation of predictive pharmacology: drug-target interaction prediction (DTI), drug-disease association prediction (DDA), and drug-target-disease association (DTD) modeling [1]. Together, these interrelated tasks provide the basis for network medicine, precision therapeutics, and drug repurposing.

This section introduces the fundamental principles of DTI, DDA, and DTD modeling. By defining each domain, describing its roles in drug discovery, and highlighting their interconnections, the discussion aims to provide conceptual clarity before delving into more advanced methods and frameworks.

1.1.1 Drug-Target Interaction (DTI) Prediction

The term "drug-target interaction" (DTI) refers to the biochemical association between a small molecule (drug) and a macromolecular entity (target), usually a protein like an enzyme, receptor, ion channel, or transporter. These interactions determine the efficacy, potency, and specificity of pharmacological interventions. Identifying novel DTIs is therefore central to early-stage drug discovery, lead optimization, toxicity assessment, and drug repositioning.

In addition to the binary prediction of whether a drug binds to a target, modern approaches often seek to estimate the binding affinity, a quantitative measure of interaction strength expressed in terms such as dissociation constant (Kd) or inhibition constant (Ki) [2]. Higher binding affinity typically indicates stronger interactions, which may translate into increased therapeutic potential. Figure 1.1 provides a schematic depiction of drug-target binding affinity, illustrating how ligands interact with their corresponding protein targets at the molecular level. Such representations emphasize the significance of quantifying not only the existence but also the strength of drug-target interactions, which is crucial for downstream drug repurposing and efficacy evaluation.

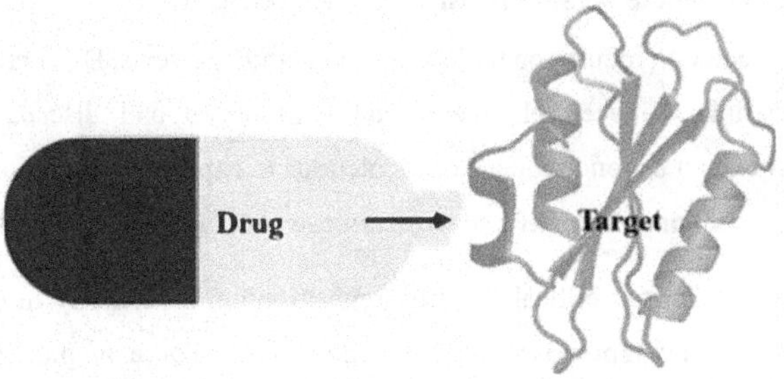

Figure 1.1: A depiction of drug target binding affinity

Historically, DTIs were identified through experimental methods such as high-throughput screening (HTS), X-ray crystallography, nuclear magnetic resonance (NMR), and affinity-based assays. While these techniques provide accurate insights, they are costly, tedious, and resource-intensive, making them infeasible for massive exploration across millions of compounds and targets.

The limitations of traditional screening have accelerated the adoption of computational techniques. Early in silico methods relied on similarity-based inference: structurally similar drugs were assumed to interact with similar targets, and conversely, homologous proteins were assumed to share binding partners. Rule-based systems, molecular docking simulations, and chemo informatics approaches provided initial predictive capabilities.

Recently, machine learning (ML) and deep learning (DL) have revolutionized DTI prediction by capturing non-linear, high-dimensional patterns. Algorithms like random forests (RF), support vector machines (SVM), and matrix factorization methods laid the foundation, while more recent architectures including recurrent neural networks (RNNs), convolutional neural networks (CNNs), and graph neural networks (GNNs), have significantly improved performance. Benchmark models such as DeepDTA, GraphDTA, and Affinity2vec exemplify the growing sophistication of computational DTI approaches.

DTI prediction not only accelerates the identification of promising compounds but also reduces costs and risks in drug development pipelines. For drug repurposing, computational DTI models allow researchers to evaluate whether approved drugs interact with novel targets, thereby enabling faster translation to clinical application.

1.1.2 Drug-Disease Association (DDA) Prediction

While DTI prediction focuses on molecular-level binding events, DDA prediction seeks to find out hidden links between pharmaceutical compounds and disease phenotypes. These associations extend beyond molecular interactions to capture therapeutic relevance whether a drug exert a beneficial effect on a specific disease condition [3].

Understanding DDAs is critical for drug repositioning, particularly in cases where existing compounds may be repurposed for new indications. For example, thalidomide, initially withdrawn due to teratogenic side effects, was later repositioned for multiple myeloma after computational and clinical evidence linked it to disease-relevant mechanisms.

Historically, DDAs were identified through clinical trials, observational studies, and post-marketing surveillance. However, the time and cost associated with such approaches are prohibitive, especially for rare diseases.

Computationally, DDA prediction leverages diverse data sources:

- Drug-related features such as chemical structures, side-effect profiles, and gene expression signatures.
- Disease-related features, including genetic mutations, dysregulated pathways, and comorbidity patterns.
- Interaction networks representing known drug-disease relationships.

Classical techniques such as matrix completion, network propagation, and collaborative filtering have been widely applied to infer missing links in drug-disease bipartite graphs. More recently, deep learning approaches using autoencoders, graph embeddings, and variational representation learning have enhanced generalization by uncovering latent structures across heterogeneous datasets.

DDA prediction contributes directly to precision medicine by stratifying patients based on molecular signatures and identifying drugs that may act on specific subtypes of a disease. This is particularly valuable in oncology and rare diseases, where traditional large-scale trials may not be feasible. By mapping drugs to disease phenotypes computationally, researchers can generate testable hypotheses for subsequent validation, significantly accelerating therapeutic discovery.

1.1.3 Drug-Target-Disease (DTD) Association Modeling

While DTI and DDA predictions provide valuable insights in isolation, therapeutic outcomes are ultimately shaped by the triadic relationship among drugs, targets, and diseases. Drug-target-disease (DTD) association modeling offers a unified framework that integrates these three domains, capturing how drugs exert clinical effects by modulating specific molecular targets within disease contexts [4].

A DTD association can be represented as a triplet of drug, target, and disease. For example, the triplet (Imatinib, BCR-ABL fusion protein, Chronic Myeloid Leukemia) captures not only the binding of Imatinib to its protein target but also its clinical relevance in treating a specific hematological cancer. DTD associations are often modeled as multi-relational graphs or knowledge tensors, where nodes represent drugs, targets, and diseases, and edges encode known or predicted relationships. To infer missing links and produce interpretable triplets, methods including tensor decomposition, graph neural networks, and knowledge graph embeddings are used. By simultaneously incorporating molecular-level interactions and phenotypic-level associations, DTD modeling provides an understanding of pharmacological activity at the systems level, polypharmacology, and off-target effects.

The ability to model DTD associations has profound implications for precision medicine. It allows researchers to:

- Identify mechanistically grounded repurposing opportunities.
- Understand drug resistance mechanisms by contextualizing target modulation in disease-specific pathways.
- Design combination therapies that target multiple nodes within disease networks.

1.1.4 Interconnections and the Closed-Loop Framework

Although DTI, DDA, and DTD prediction are often studied independently, they are best understood as interconnected tasks forming a closed-loop system in predictive pharmacology.

- DTI prediction identifies candidate molecular interactions.
- DDA prediction determines the potential disease contexts where these interactions may have therapeutic relevance.
- DTD modeling integrates both dimensions, linking molecular interactions to clinical outcomes.

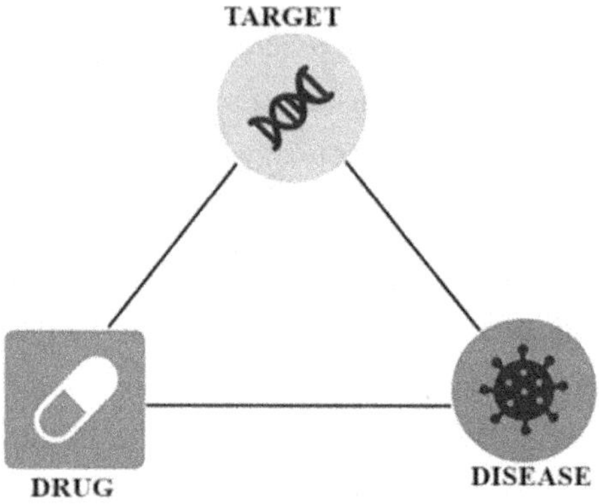

Figure 1.2: Drug Target Disease Association

This closed-loop perspective enables bidirectional knowledge flow: novel DTIs can suggest potential DDAs, while disease-centric insights can guide the search for previously overlooked DTIs. Together, these domains create a virtuous cycle that accelerates drug discovery and repurposing.

A schematic representation (Figure 1.2) often depicts drugs, targets, and diseases as vertices of a triangle, with edges representing pairwise interactions (DTI and DDA) and the full triplet representing DTD associations. This conceptual diagram highlights how individual predictions connect to form a comprehensive map of therapeutic relationships.

1.2 Background

The rapid evolution of computational biology and bioinformatics has created new opportunities in drug discovery and development [5]. With the increasing availability of large-scale biological, chemical, and clinical datasets, computational methods have become central to understanding the complex interplay among drugs, their molecular targets, and disease phenotypes [6]. Within this landscape, predictive modeling has advanced considerably, evolving from heuristic and rule-based methods to sophisticated deep learning and graph-based frameworks.

At the molecular level, drug efficacy and specificity are largely governed by the interactions between chemical compounds and their biological targets, typically proteins such as enzymes, receptors, or transporters [7]. Experimental techniques, including high-throughput screening, X-ray crystallography, and affinity assays, have traditionally been the gold standard for identifying drug-target interactions (DTIs). While effective, these approaches are resource-intensive and costly. In contrast, computational methods provide scalable and cost-effective alternatives by leveraging commonalities in existing interaction data [8].

Early computational strategies for DTI prediction were primarily similarity- and rule-based, drawing on chemical descriptors, protein sequence features, and interaction profiles. Classical ML models, such as SVMs, random forests, and matrix factorization techniques, laid the foundation for predictive pharmacology. These methods demonstrated the feasibility of exploiting feature representations to identify novel DTIs, though they were limited by linear assumptions and restricted scalability. Over time, computational DTI modeling has progressed toward ML and DL paradigms, which are capable of capturing non-linear, high-dimensional relationships within biological data [9-11].

Modern approaches now utilize rich descriptors of molecular structures, protein sequences, and interaction networks, with chemical substructures encoded as molecular fingerprints and protein characteristics represented through amino acid composition, physicochemical properties, or sequence embeddings [12].

These methods established the feasibility of exploiting feature representations to predict novel DTIs, though they were often constrained by linear assumptions and limited scalability.

The recent paradigm shift to deep learning, introduced models that have the ability to immediately learn intricate, nonlinear patterns from molecular and biological data. CNNs and RNNs were first employed to model drug and protein sequences, followed by GNNs, which provided a natural representation of molecular structures and heterogeneous biological networks [13,14]. Models such as DeepDTA [15], GraphDTA [16], and Affinity2vec [17] have demonstrated the benefits of using end-to-end learning to predict binding affinity and achieve cutting-edge results on standardized datasets. These advances enhance forecast accuracy and expand the discovery space for novel chemical scaffolds, polypharmacology, and resistance mechanisms.

Building on the success of DTI modeling, drug-disease association (DDA) prediction has emerged as a complementary domain, leveraging heterogeneous biomedical data to identify therapeutic opportunities beyond known indications [18,19]. Systems biology and network pharmacology frameworks exploit similarities among drugs (chemical structure, side effects), diseases (gene expression, comorbidity), and known associations to uncover novel links [20]. Computational strategies have evolved from matrix completion, label propagation, and network-based inference [21,22] to more advanced approaches based on autoencoders, variational embeddings, and knowledge graph representations [23,24]. Incorporating resources such as LINCS, GEO, and DisGeNET has enabled multi-view learning and graph-based fusion, yielding improved generalization across diverse therapeutic contexts [25,26].

The natural extension of these domains is drug-target-disease (DTD) association modeling, which integrates drug, protein, and disease information into a unified predictive framework. Representations such as multi-relational graphs and tensors capture tripartite interactions, while techniques including knowledge graph embeddings and tensor factorization allow for scalable link prediction across biomedical entities [27–29]. This triadic modeling approach offers mechanistic insights into how drugs modulate disease phenotypes through specific targets, thus advancing drug repositioning and systems-level therapeutics.

As the field progresses, DTD modeling has gained particular traction in oncology, where cancer's inherent heterogeneity demands integrative strategies. Multi-omics datasets from resources such as TCGA, ICGC, and CPTAC provide transcriptomic, genomic, epigenomic, and proteomic features that enable precision stratification of cancer subtypes [30]. Machine learning approaches that fuse heterogeneous modalities via multi-view learning, attention mechanisms, and heterogeneous GNNs are capable of encoding the intricate relationships among genes, pathways, drugs, and disease states [31-34]. These integrative methods reveal novel DTD associations with translational potential for biomarker discovery, drug repurposing, and combination therapy design.

Despite substantial progress, several challenges remain unresolved. Data imbalance continues to hinder predictive accuracy and robustness, particularly for rare diseases and under-studied targets. Binding affinity models must contend with dynamic protein-ligand interactions and the influence of microenvironmental variability. Knowledge graphs, while powerful, require effective strategies for prioritizing candidates under sparse prior knowledge. Recent efforts toward neuro-symbolic AI, integrating neural representation learning with symbolic reasoning, hold promise for addressing these gaps [33]. By enabling both predictive power and mechanistic interpretability, such approaches could accelerate the rational design of therapies in precision oncology and rare disease contexts [34-37].

Thus, this dissertation seeks to advance the field by addressing the following research questions:

- Can hybrid deep learning frameworks overcome data imbalance and structural limitations to predict DTIs with higher accuracy and lower false-positive rates than state-of-the-art methods?
- How can binding affinity prediction models account for dynamic protein-ligand interactions and microenvironmental variability without relying on 3D structural data?
- Can knowledge graphs systematically prioritize repurposing candidates for rare diseases and heterogeneous cancers, even with sparse prior knowledge?
- Is it feasible to integrate multi-omics data into neuro-symbolic models to predict cancer-specific therapeutic targets with explainable mechanistic insights?

1.3 Motivation

The traditional drug discovery pipeline is a time-intensive and cost-prohibitive process, typically requiring over 10-15 years and an investment exceeding $2 billion to bring a new compound from initial screening to clinical approval. Despite significant advances in high-throughput screening and molecular profiling, the failure rate remains alarmingly high, particularly in the later stages of development due to unforeseen toxicity or insufficient efficacy. This inefficiency underscores the need for more predictive, data-driven methodologies that can systematically reduce the risk, cost, and time associated with therapeutic development.

Figure 1.3. explains traditional vs. computational drug discovery pipelines. The traditional process relies on high-throughput screening, lead optimization, and preclinical/clinical trials, whereas computational approaches leverage knowledge graphs and deep learning-based drug-target interaction prediction, virtual screening, and experimental validation, thereby reducing time, cost, and failure rates.

By utilizing current medications with established pharmacokinetic and safety profiles for novel disease indications, drug repurposing has become a very viable substitute. By bypassing several early-phase trials, repurposing not only accelerates the drug development timeline but also significantly reduces associated costs and regulatory hurdles. However, successful repurposing requires a deep understanding of the mechanistic links between drugs, their molecular targets, and disease-specific pathophysiology, an area where computational modeling can play a transformative role.

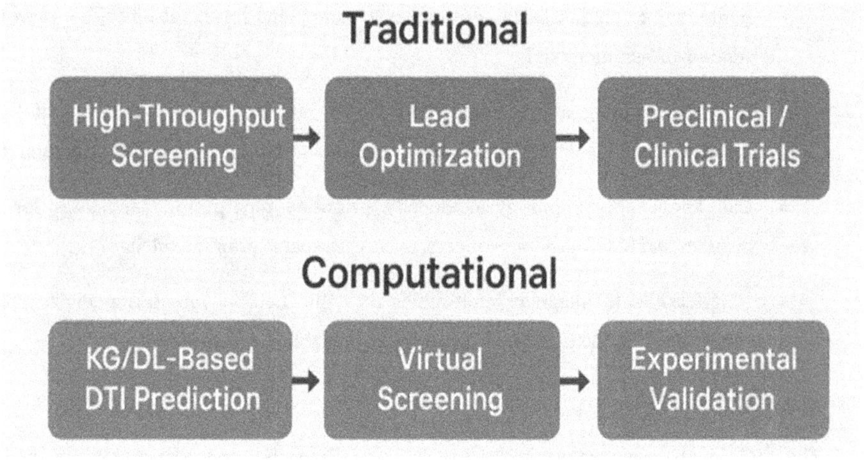

Figure 1.3: Illustration of traditional and computational processes

Moreover, the dynamic nature of disease biology, especially in complex and heterogeneous disorders like cancer, introduces the challenge of target adaptability. Molecular targets often exhibit context-dependent behaviors, altered expression patterns, or mutational escape mechanisms, necessitating predictive models that can adapt to biological variability and uncover latent drug-target-disease relationships.

The convergence of large-scale bioinformatics resources, graph-based learning, and multi-omics data integration offers a powerful foundation to address these challenges. By building intelligent systems that learn from existing pharmacological, genomic, and clinical data, it becomes possible to identify novel targets, stratify disease subtypes, and prioritize repurposable drugs with high translational potential. This research is motivated by the urgent need to develop such scalable, interpretable, and biologically grounded frameworks for accelerating therapeutic discovery in a cost-effective and precision-oriented manner.

1.4 Scope of the Research

The scope of this research lies at the intersection of artificial intelligence (AI) and translational pharmacology, aiming to redefine the computational landscape for drug discovery and therapeutic development. The work addresses persistent inefficiencies in traditional and modern drug discovery approaches, ranging from limited chemical and biological space exploration to the inability of current models to generalize across imbalanced or sparse datasets, particularly in rare diseases and precision oncology. This thesis focuses on three core problem domains: identifying robust drug-target interactions, repurposing known drugs for novel diseases, and predicting context-specific therapeutic targets in complex diseases like cancer. The study encompasses the development of deep learning and graph-based computational frameworks that integrate sequence data, molecular structures, knowledge graphs, and multi-omics datasets to offer biologically grounded, interpretable insights.

The research is designed to utilize publicly available biomedical databases, spanning drug-target pairs, disease associations, omics profiles, and structured knowledge networks. Emphasis is placed on data imbalance, lack of annotations for rare disease pathways, and heterogeneity in cancer subtypes, three major barriers to generalizable, scalable computational solutions. This study is restricted to computational (in silico) predictions and validations using curated datasets. While experimental wet-lab validation is beyond its scope, the findings are contextualized and supported by evidence from clinically validated case studies. Geographically, the research adopts a global approach by utilizing international datasets such as KIBA, DrugBank, DisGeNET, and TCGA.

Temporally, the models are designed to be future-proof and scalable, enabling continuous learning as new biological and clinical data become available. Once the key challenges in each domain are addressed, this research aims to contribute optimized, interpretable, and clinically relevant AI-driven frameworks. These contributions are expected to support more precise drug development strategies, reduce attrition in clinical pipelines, and unlock therapeutic options for underexplored diseases.

1.5 Problem Statement and Research Objectives

1.5.1 Problem Statement

Use advanced computational methodologies, specifically deep learning-based frameworks, to accurately predict drug-target interactions, systematically leverage knowledge networks for drug repurposing, and identify novel cancer-specific therapeutic targets through multi-omics data integration, thereby enhancing the efficiency and efficacy of the drug discovery and development process.

1.5.2 Research Objectives

- Develop an automated, optimized deep learning-based DTI (drug target interactions) prediction that can handle data imbalance issues and enhance prediction accuracy.
- Leverage knowledge networks to facilitate drug repurposing, aiming to systematically identify and validate novel therapeutic applications for existing drugs, thereby enhancing drug discovery and development processes.
- Implement a deep learning-based methodology for the prediction of novel therapeutic targets specific to distinct cancer types, leveraging multi-omics data integration

1.5.3 Proposed Methodology

The methodology is structured as a cascading computational pipeline that progresses from DTI prediction to drug-disease association inference and culminates in context-aware, cancer-specific drug-disease-target interaction modeling. Each component addresses critical gaps in conventional approaches while ensuring interpretability, scalability, and biological relevance. Figure 1.4 illustrates the workflow.

This sequential approach is designed to optimize drug-target interaction analysis, exploit knowledge networks for drug repurposing, and integrate multi-omics data for precise target discovery in oncology.

➤ **Objective 1: Designing an Optimized Deep Learning Framework for Drug-Target Interaction (DTI) Prediction**

The study initiates by addressing the core challenge of predicting DTI with higher precision, scalability, and fairness, particularly in the presence of class imbalance, which frequently skews predictions toward dominant classes.

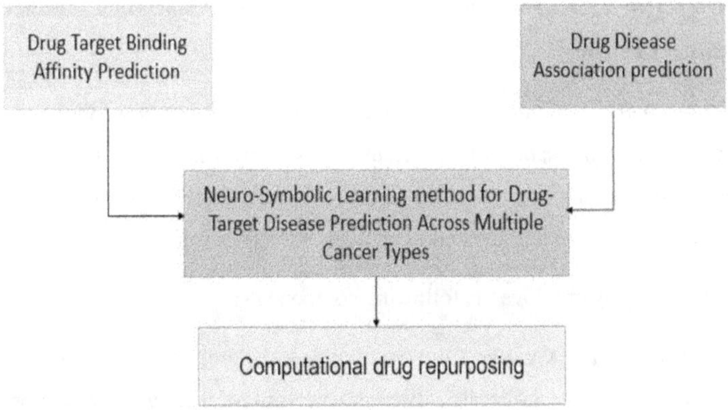

Figure 1.4: Workflow of the computational drug discovery process

To this end, two alternative techniques are explored in parallel:

- **Approach A** - Drug Target Interaction (DTI) Identification Using HBO nature-inspired metaheuristic optimization algorithm. Leveraging the explorative and exploitative capabilities of the Honey Badger Optimization algorithm, DTI prediction is reframed as a global search task over molecular features. Here, encoded representations of drug SMILES strings and protein sequences are processed through feature extractors (1D-CNN), and HBO is utilized to select optimal feature subsets and decision thresholds. This improves model generalizability and reduces noise, particularly from false positives arising in unbalanced datasets.
- **Approach B** - LAMB Optimizer for binding affinity Modeling. In a complementary stream, a deep learning regression model is trained to predict binding affinity values using a Transformer-Conv1D hybrid, optimized using the Layer-wise Adaptive Moments optimizer for batch training. LAMB, known for its ability to converge on large batch sizes without compromising model stability, enables faster learning across skewed data distributions. This addresses class imbalance not by reweighting the data, but by stabilizing gradient updates during training.

These two paths are subjected to comparative evaluation, based on AUC, PR-AUC, F1-score, and performance on rare drug-target pairs. The goal is to determine whether evolutionary metaheuristics or optimizer-level innovations are better suited for tackling class imbalance while preserving predictive power.

➤ **Objective 2: Knowledge-Driven Drug-Disease Association Prediction via Graph Attention Learning**

Building upon the reliable DTI predictions from the first phase, the work transitions into discovering new therapeutic applications through network-informed repurposing. Here, drug-disease associations are modelled using a hybrid framework that integrates biomedical knowledge graphs with graph neural network (GNN) learning.

The methodology employs the following components:

- **Knowledge Graph Construction:** A heterogeneous graph is constructed by integrating drug-disease, disease-gene, drug-target, and protein-protein interaction datasets. These relations are enriched with ontological annotations (e.g., MeSH terms, GO terms), ensuring biomedical relevance.
- **Drug-Disease Prediction using Graph Attention Network (GAT):** A Graph Attention Network is then applied to dynamically weigh the neighborhood influence of drugs and diseases in the latent embedding space. The GAT learns task-specific attention scores, ensuring that only the most relevant interactions contribute to the prediction of novel associations.

This stage uncovers hidden links in the biomedical network that may suggest alternative indications for existing compounds. Such predictions are ranked using statistical confidence scores and further validated through literature mining and existing clinical evidence.

➤ **Objective 3: Cancer-Specific Target Identification Using Multi-Omics and Neuro-Symbolic Learning**

The final and most integrative segment of the study focuses on precise therapeutic target discovery in cancer, leveraging multi-omics data and explainable neuro-symbolic models. The steps include:

- **Multi-Omics Data Assembly:** Omics layers, including gene expression, degree centrality, and page score, as well as DNA methylation and mutation profiles, are collected for chosen cancer types based on the TCGA (Cancer Genome Atlas) and GEO.
- **Feature Integration:** A custom pipeline integrates omics layers, generating unified

embeddings that represent the functional state of genes per sample. Known gene-drug, gene-disease, and gene-feature associations are mapped over these representations.

- **Neuro-Symbolic Prediction Framework:** A novel Neuro-Symbolic model is employed, wherein a deep neural network extracts latent features, while a symbolic reasoning engine is layered above to derive interpretable associations between drugs, diseases, and target genes, thereby enabling explainable predictions and enhancing biological insight for therapeutic discovery

This framework achieves two-fold objectives: it identifies novel cancer-specific therapeutic targets and provides biologically explainable insights into their mechanisms, bridging the gap between AI predictions and clinician trust, thereby enhancing precision oncology and accelerating translational biomedical research outcomes.

1.6 Dissertation Chapter Outline

Chapter 1: Introduction

This chapter introduces the fundamental concepts of drug discovery, DTIs, and the challenges posed by traditional experimental methods. It emphasizes the importance of deep learning, and knowledge networks in addressing drug discovery bottlenecks. The chapter concludes with the research motivation, identified research gaps, scope of the research, problem statement, objectives, and proposed methodology.

Chapter 2: Review of Literature

This chapter provides a thorough review of the current state of research on drug repurposing, therapeutic target discovery with AI, and DTI prediction. It discusses traditional and modern machine learning methods, limitations of structure-based models, current data imbalance solutions, the rise of graph-based knowledge networks, and the role of multi-omics integration in precision medicine. Critical gaps in generalization, interpretability, and systematic drug repurposing are identified to justify the proposed methodologies.

Chapter 3: Datasets And Resources for the Proposed Methodology

This Chapter presents the datasets and resources underpinning the proposed methodology. It details benchmark datasets for drug-target interaction prediction, knowledge network datasets for drug repurposing, and the development of a novel multi-omics dataset, OncoOmicsNet, for cancer target prediction. The chapter outlines dataset sources, structure, preprocessing, and their alignment with each research objective.

Chapter 4: Optimized Deep Learning Framework for Drug-Target Interaction Prediction

This chapter addresses the issue of data imbalance and prediction inefficiencies in DTI prediction by proposing and evaluating two advanced computational strategies. This study explores drug-target interaction (DTI) prediction using two advanced optimization methods. First, the Honey Badger Optimization (HBO) algorithm is used for identifying DTIs through binary classification, especially on imbalanced datasets. Next, the Layer-wise Adaptive Moments (LAMB) optimizer is applied to predict DTBA using a regression model, designed to handle noisy biochemical data. Finally, a comparative analysis is performed between the HBO-based classifier and the LAMB-based regressor using performance measures such as ROC-AUC, F1-score, recall, precision, and prediction error to determine the more effective approach.

Chapter 5: Drug Repurposing via Knowledge Networks using Graph-Based Deep Learning

This chapter presents a systematic approach to drug repurposing using graph-based methods. It first builds a knowledge graph by integrating data on drugs, diseases, targets, pathways, and side effects. Then, it introduces a hybrid graph attention network model that uses graph embeddings and attention mechanisms to predict new drug-disease associations. Finally, it validates the model through case studies and explores potential treatments for rare cancers.

Chapter 6: Multi-Omics and Neuro-Symbolic Learning for Novel Target Discovery in Cancer

This chapter presents a deep learning and symbolic reasoning framework for predicting cancer-specific therapeutic targets. It integrates and processes multi-omics data (like gene expression and mutations) for cancers such as breast, lung, colon, and bladder. The model combines neural networks with rule-based AI to provide interpretable predictions about drug sensitivity and target likelihood.

Chapter 7: Conclusion and Future Work

Summarizes the contributions of each chapter and how they address the identified research gaps. The chapter also presents a quantitative summary of results achieved, discusses the practical implications for computational drug discovery, and outlines potential directions for future research, such as incorporating real-time patient data, improving symbolic reasoning, or validating predictions through in vitro assays.

CHAPTER 2

LITERATURE REVIEW

2.1 Introduction

The intersection of AI and drug discovery has catalysed a paradigm shift in the way therapeutic compounds are identified, repurposed, and personalized. Traditional drug development pipelines, often constrained by time, cost, and experimental limitations, are increasingly being supplemented by data-driven approaches that leverage ML, DL, and network-based models. Within this broader landscape, three critical challenges persist: predicting drug-target interactions (DTIs) with high fidelity, identifying novel drug-disease associations for drug repurposing, and integrating multi-omics data to pinpoint disease-specific targets. This literature review explores each of these dimensions, focusing on the methodologies, datasets, and research gaps relevant to the objectives of this study.

The first objective revolves around the precise forecast of DTBA, a fundamental aspect of understanding molecular interactions. Classical computational techniques, such as molecular docking, often fall short due to their dependence on structural data and high computational costs. In contrast, ML and DL models are emerging as strong alternatives by learning interaction patterns from large-scale biochemical data [15]. These models utilize various forms of data encoding, such as amino acid sequences for proteins and SMILES representation for drug compounds and architectures like CNNs, RNNs, and Transformers to enhance predictive performance. However, challenges such as class imbalance, overfitting, and lack of interpretability still hinder real-world deployment.

The second objective expands the scope by focusing on drug repurposing through knowledge-driven drug-disease association modelling. Biomedical knowledge networks, which integrate diverse sources such as protein-protein, gene-disease and drug-target interaction data, offer a rich context for uncovering latent therapeutic relationships [29,36] GNNs, specifically Graph Attention Networks (GATs), have been successfully applied to these heterogeneous graphs, enabling context-aware learning and improved association prediction. Despite promising results, many studies are limited by incomplete knowledge graphs, non-biological noise in the network, and limited validation using clinical evidence.

The third objective of this study builds upon the first two by targeting context-aware therapeutic modeling in oncology. Cancer, being a complex and heterogeneous disease, necessitates multi-dimensional modeling of genomic, transcriptomic, and epigenomic data. Multi-omics integration has gained momentum in recent years with the advent of publicly available resources like TCGA and GEO [37,38]. Integrative models aim to capture the dynamic interplay of genetic alterations, expression levels, and regulatory mechanisms to identify precise targets. Here, neuro-symbolic learning frameworks are gaining interest as they blend the predictive neural network skills combined with symbolic reasoning's explainability, a key requirement in clinical decision support.

This literature study aims to systematically analyze existing research along these three objectives. Each section presents a focused discussion on representative models, benchmarking datasets, evaluation strategies, and observed limitations. Particular attention is paid to recent innovations, such as nature-inspired metaheuristics, advanced optimizers like LAMB, and the use of biomedical ontologies in graph construction. The chapter concludes with a synthesis of findings and a critical analysis of research gaps, thereby motivating the need for an integrated, cascading pipeline as proposed in this thesis.

2.2 Review on Drug-Target Interaction (DTI) and Binding Affinity Prediction

DTI prediction is essential to modern drug discovery, as it helps identify potential therapeutic candidates and understand adverse effects by determining which drugs bind to which biological targets. Binding affinity represents the quantitative strength of this interaction, providing critical insights into drug efficacy and dosage. Traditionally, DTIs were identified using wet-lab methods such as high-throughput screening or molecular docking, which are tedious and costly. To overcome these limitations, computational techniques, especially ML and DL, have emerged as efficient alternatives, offering high scalability and being able to learn from intrinsic biological data patterns [39–41].

Before the rise of machine learning, DTIs were primarily predicted using molecular docking, ligand-based screening and quantitative structure-activity relationship (QSAR) models. These physics- and chemistry-driven methods required detailed 3D structural information of both targets and drugs, limiting their applicability to well-characterised molecules [42,43].

Additionally, docking simulations are computationally expensive and often fail to generalize across diverse protein families. QSAR and ligand-based models, while faster, suffer from poor scalability and limited accuracy on novel compounds [44]. These constraints have catalyzed a paradigm shift toward data-driven approaches, where ML and DL techniques offer scalable, structure-agnostic solutions for learning complex biological interactions directly from raw data [45]. Early computational strategies for DTI prediction predominantly employed traditional ML methods. Yamanishi et al. [46] were among the first to frame DTI prediction as a binary classification problem, utilizing similarity-based models to integrate genomic space (targets) and chemical space (drugs) into a compact representation. Extending this approach, Ezzat et.al [22] and Cheng et al. [47] employed kernel-based regression models that leveraged chemical and genomic similarities, significantly enhancing the ability to predict interactions for previously unseen drug-target pairings.

ability to predict interactions for previously unseen drug-target pairs.

To address data imbalance and improve generalizability, Ezzat et al. [22] proposed ensemble-based models such as Gradient Boosting and Random Forests. These models demonstrated improved performance by combining diverse classifiers and incorporating handcrafted features like molecular fingerprints and amino acid compositions. In addition, the authors introduced graph-regularized matrix factorization (GRMF) methods to capture the low-dimensional nonlinear manifolds inherent in drug-target interaction data. By integrating graph-based regularization, their framework effectively modeled the structural dependencies within the interaction network, particularly enhancing predictions for "orphan" drugs and targets. Their results underscored the importance of graph-aware ensemble approaches in mitigating data sparsity, class imbalance, and cold-start challenges prevalent in DTI prediction tasks.

Keum and Nam [48] introduced SELF-BLM, a hybrid framework that integrates self-training support vector machines (SVM) with bipartite local models (BLM) for enhanced drug-target interaction (DTI) prediction. Unlike conventional BLM approaches that tend to classify unknown interactions as negative, SELF-BLM employs a clustering-based strategy to effectively separate unlabeled interactions from true negatives. These unlabeled interactions are subsequently refined through self-training, leading to more robust local classification models. When evaluated across four key protein families, enzymes, ion channels, nuclear receptors, and G-protein coupled receptors (GPCRs), the method consistently demonstrated superior performance, accurately identifying both validated and novel potential interactions.

In parallel, Pahikkala et al. [49] argued that rethinking the formulation of DTI prediction tasks by modeling them as ranking or regression problems rather than binary classification could yield deeper insights, particularly in understanding binding affinities rather than just the presence or absence of interaction. They emphasized that overly simplified binary formulations often fail to capture the inherent complexity of drug-target relationships in real-world pharmacological contexts. The study further highlighted that factors such as dataset composition, evaluation procedures, and experimental settings can significantly influence prediction outcomes, thereby leading to overly optimistic or misleading conclusions. By advocating for more rigorous evaluation methodologies, including nested cross-validation and careful separation of drugs and targets between training and test sets, the authors provided critical guidelines to enhance the reliability and realism of DTI studies. Their work thus underscored the need for benchmarking datasets and evaluation practices that more accurately reflect the continuous and multifaceted nature of drug-target interactions.

Despite the foundational contributions of these classical ML approaches, their performance eventually plateaued due to reliance on manually engineered features and limited capacity for complex pattern recognition. These limitations paved the way for more expressive DL models, which could automatically extract sophisticated characteristics from raw data and better capture the underlying biological complexities [40].

To overcome the shortcomings of traditional ML, recent years have witnessed a paradigm shift toward DL based models for DTI and binding affinity prediction. These methods eliminate manual feature engineering by learning directly from raw representations of protein sequences and drug molecules, enabling the capture of intricate patterns and nonlinear dependencies.

Binding affinity prediction models primarily frame the task as a regression problem to estimate continuous biochemical values such as Kd, Ki, and IC50, offering more informative insights compared to binary classification. Pahikkala et al. introduced KronRLS, a kernel-based regression approach that effectively models continuous binding scores [49].

He et.al [50] proposed SimBoost, a gradient boosting model utilizing similarity-based features, which achieved high accuracy in estimating binding affinities. Öztürk et al. [15] introduced

DeepDTA, a pioneering deep learning framework that predicts drug-target binding affinities directly from sequence information of drugs and proteins. Unlike prior approaches that relied on 3D structural data or handcrafted 2D molecular features, DeepDTA employs CNNs to extract high-level representations from one-dimensional sequences. This methodological shift enabled the model to effectively capture underlying biochemical interaction patterns without requiring complex structural preprocessing. Experimental evaluations demonstrated that DeepDTA consistently outperformed established methods such as KronRLS and SimBoost across benchmark datasets, achieving superior Concordance Index (CI) scores. These findings established DeepDTA as a cornerstone model in the advancement of DL based DTI prediction.

Building on this, Karimi et al. introduced DeepAffinity, a semi-supervised DL framework that integrates convolutional and recurrent NN to jointly encode compound and protein representations directly from sequences. Using both labeled and unlabeled data, the model effectively captures complex sequence-structure relationships while improving generalization to unseen protein classes. Importantly, the incorporation of separate and joint attention mechanisms enabled the model to highlight biologically meaningful interaction regions, thereby enhancing interpretability alongside predictive accuracy. Furthermore, the study explored transfer learning and alternative graph-based representations, demonstrating the robustness and adaptability of DeepAffinity for diverse drug discovery scenarios [51].

Tsubaki et al. proposed a more expressive end-to-end model by combining graph neural networks (GNNs) for drug molecular graphs and CNNs for protein sequences. Their architecture integrated attention mechanisms to identify interaction-specific protein regions and was particularly effective on imbalanced datasets [52].

Manica et al. further extended this direction by presenting a multimodal attention-based convolutional encoder tailored for interpretable anticancer drug sensitivity prediction. Their architecture integrates compound structures (via SMILES), tumor gene expression profiles and previous information from networks of protein-protein interactions. Utilizing multiscale convolution and attention, the model enhances interpretability and generalizability for precision oncology and de novo drug design [53].

Bae and Nam introduced GraphATT-DTA, a novel attention-based framework that captures interactions between drug substructures and protein subsequences that range from local to global. This model significantly outperformed prior methods on datasets like Davis and

Binding DB, leveraging attention for both predictive accuracy and interpretability of binding sites [54].

In parallel, Bagherian et al. discussed critical challenges in DTI modeling, including data imbalance, incomplete labeling, interpretability constraints, and poor generalization. They emphasized the necessity for biological validation, integration of diverse omics data, and standardized benchmarks to improve real-world applicability [45].

Complementing architectural innovations, Cheng et al. proposed hybrid multi-view frameworks that integrate chemical, genomic, pathway, and disease-related information. These approaches aim to enhance both prediction accuracy and drug repurposing capabilities in multi-objective settings [55].

Collectively, these deep learning-based methods have laid a robust foundation for next-generation drug discovery tools, with demonstrated applications in optimizing kinase inhibitors in oncology and developing antivirals for diseases like COVID-19 and influenza.

Despite the promising performance of ML and DL approaches in DTI and binding affinity prediction, several challenges remain. DL models, in particular, are susceptible to overfitting on smaller or unbalanced datasets and frequently lack interpretability, making it difficult to glean physiologically significant conclusions. The scarcity of high-quality, labeled DTI data further limits training efficacy. Moreover, current models often struggle with generalization across multiple protein families, reducing their applicability in broader drug discovery pipelines. These limitations underscore critical research gaps, particularly in designing interpretable, data-efficient, and generalizable models, which are discussed are avenues for future innovation.

Objective 1 aims to enhance DTI prediction by overcoming class imbalance and improving precision. Compared to traditional ML models reliant on handcrafted features, deep learning (DL) offers superior representation learning but faces overfitting and instability. To address this, two hybrid DL methods are explored: HBO-driven feature optimization to reduce false positives, and a Transformer-Conv1D model optimized using LAMB for stable training on imbalanced data. These approaches exploit DL's strength in learning complex patterns while integrating optimization strategies to boost robustness and fairness, key to scalable, high-accuracy DTI prediction.

Table 2.1: Summary of DTI and Binding Affinity Prediction Methods

Category	Method/Model	Key Features	Advantages	Limitations
Traditional	Molecular Docking [42,43]	Physics-based simulation of drug binding	Accurate for known 3D structures	Time-consuming, structure-dependent
	Ligand-Based Screening [56]	Similarity search with known ligands	Fast & simple	Poor generalization to novel compounds
	QSAR Models [47]	Statistical relationship between structure and activity	Interpretable	Limited scalability, manual feature engineering
Traditional ML	Similarity-Based Classification [46]	Integrates chemical and genomic similarity	First binary DTI classifier	Limited to known interactions
	Kernel-Based Regression [47]	Regression using drug-target similarities	Predicts continuous scores	Feature engineering required
	Ensemble Models [22]	Random Forest, Gradient Boosting, handcrafted features	Handles class imbalance, good performance	Interpretability trade-offs
	SELF-BLM (Self-training Bipartite Local Model) [48]	Uses clustering to differentiate unlabeled and negative interactions	outperforms standard BLM in most protein classes	Limited capacity to learn complex hierarchical patterns and poor generalisation.
	KronRLS [49]	Kernel regression for binding scores	Handles regression for binding affinity	Needs kernel design
	SimBoost [50]	Gradient boosting with similarity features	Good regression performance	Still relies on engineered features
Deep Learning	DeepDTA [15]	1D CNNs for SMILES and sequences	No manual features, good benchmarks	Limited interpretability
	DeepAffinity [51]	Attention-based CNNs	Highlights key regions, better insights	Complexity increases
	GNN + CNN + Attention [52]	GNNs for drugs, CNNs for proteins	Captures structural and sequential info	Imbalanced data issues
	Multimodal Encoder [53]	Combines SMILES, gene expression, and PPI	High interpretability, multi-source data	Requires large annotated data

	GraphATT-DTA [54]	Attention on drug substructures and protein sub-sequences	High accuracy & interpretability	Complexity & training cost
Deep Learning	Hybrid Multi-View Models [55]	Integration of pathway, omics, disease data	Better repurposing and accuracy	Complex design, integration issues

2.3 Review on Knowledge-Driven Drug-Disease Association Prediction via Graph-Based Learning Approaches

Drug repurposing, the process of identifying novel therapeutic applications for existing drugs, provides a reasonable and time-saving technique in drug discovery. Traditional approaches often miss latent associations between drugs and diseases, especially for rare conditions. In recent years, data-driven knowledge networks have emerged as a powerful foundation for drug-disease association (DDA) prediction by integrating diverse biomedical relationships. To fully harness this potential, there is a growing need for scalable, interpretable, and integrative AI models, notably graph-based approaches like GNNs, GATs, and biomedical knowledge graphs (KGs).

Zitnik et al. [36] laid the groundwork for using graphs to model intricate biomedical systems, where nodes denote entities such as genes, diseases, targets, or drugs and edges encode relationships like chemical similarity, genetic interactions, or known disease associations. This representation facilitates relational reasoning by capturing direct and indirect links in biological networks. Unlike flat feature vectors, graphs encode multi-relational and topological information, enabling the discovery of novel DDAs through topological proximity and shared neighborhoods. Techniques such as Random Walk with Restart [57] and Network Propagation [58] have been used to diffuse signals across nodes, thereby ranking potential disease candidates for a given drug. However, these approaches often rely on handcrafted similarity metrics and cannot generalize well to unseen entities, motivating the shift toward learned representations via graph neural models.

Biomedical Knowledge Graphs (KGs) represent entities such as diseases, genes, drugs, and proteins as nodes and edges in a graph. These heterogeneous graphs integrate multi-modal data, molecular, clinical, and pharmacological, and unify information from diverse databases using ontologies. This structured representation enables machine-readable reasoning and supports knowledge-driven drug repurposing predictions.

Himmelstein et al. introduced Hetionet, a comprehensive KG integrating data from 29 sources, including DrugBank, DisGeNET, and Disease Ontology, to uncover novel drug-disease relationships using a metapath-based approach. Their model successfully predicted therapeutic use cases like bupropion for nicotine dependence with experimental validation, demonstrating the predictive power of cross-domain integration [59].

Wang et al. developed COVID-KG, a real-time updated knowledge graph comprising chemical, biological, and clinical data to accelerate COVID-19 drug repurposing. Their graph-based framework used path ranking algorithms to prioritize candidate drugs, identifying baricitinib and remdesivir as potential antivirals [60].

Gao et al. presented a computational framework, KG-Predict, that constructs a knowledge graph (GP-KG) by integrating multiple phenotypic and genotypic databases. KG-Predict collects heterogeneous topological and semantic information to acquire low-dimensional representations of objects and connections, enabling the inference of new drug-disease interactions. Applied to Alzheimer's disease, KG-Predict highlighted both active clinical and FDA-approved trials for anti-AD medicines, demonstrating its effectiveness in drug repurposing [61].

Yan et.al proposed that for the repurposing of drugs, Adaptive Multi-View Learning (AMVL) combines large language model (LLM) representations, knowledge graph embeddings, and chemical-induced transcriptional profiles (CTPs). By fusing heterogeneous data via ensemble optimization and matrix factorization, AMVL achieved cutting edge performance across multiple datasets and showed strong literature-backed predictive capabilities [62].

Olasunkanmi et al. proposed EDGAR (Explainable Enrichment-Driven Graph Reasoner), a link prediction framework for large-scale biomedical KGs. EDGAR infers new edges by mining entity-local rules through enrichment analysis, providing inherently explainable and statistically significant inference results. Applied to the ROBOKOP KG for Alzheimer's disease, EDGAR identified 1,246 additional drug candidates, with the top 10 validated using medical literature evidence [63]. Gharizadeh et al. introduced HGTDR (Heterogeneous Graph Transformer for Drug Repurposing), a three-step approach involving the construction of a heterogeneous KG, utilization of a heterogeneous graph transformer network, and computation of relationship scores. HGTDR demonstrated comparable performance to previous methods and was validated through medical studies, showcasing its capability to predict drug-protein and disease-protein interrelations [64].

Toonsi et al. developed a Causal Knowledge Graph (CKG) framework that extends traditional KGs with formal causal semantics, enabling principled causal inference. By developing a drug-disease CKG that incorporates illness development pathways, drug indications, and side effects, they applied mediation analysis to identify adverse drug effects. Their method found previously unreported significant candidate side effects and successfully replicated known adverse medication reactions[65].

KGML-xDTD, a knowledge graph-based ML framework for explainably predicting drug-disease associations, was proposed by Ma et al.. The framework not only predicts treatment probabilities but also provides biological explanations via KG path-based mechanisms of action. Applied to various datasets, KGML-xDTD achieved cutting-edge performance in both predictions and summary of medication MOA pathways selected by humans [66] .

This framework identifies novel cancer-specific therapeutic targets and provides biologically explainable insights, bridging AI predictions and clinician trust to enhance precision oncology, translational research, and evidence-based clinical decision-making.

Zitnik et al. introduced Decagon, a pioneering model that employs Graph Convolutional Networks (GCNs) to forecast polypharmacy adverse effects through modeling a multimodal graph comprising protein-protein interactions, drug-target interactions, and drug-drug interactions. Decagon demonstrated the capability of GCNs to handle multirelational data, achieving significant improvements over traditional methods [36].

The GraphDPA model utilized GCNs to represent drugs and pathways within a unified graph structure. This approach enabled the effective prediction of drug-pathway associations, highlighting the versatility of GCNs in various biomedical contexts [67].

The HINGRL model creates a diverse knowledge network that incorporates protein-disease, drug-protein, and drug-disease relationships. By applying graph representation learning techniques, HINGRL effectively predicts new drug indications, emphasizing the importance of biological context in DDA prediction [68].

HEDDI-Net, proposed by researchers in 2024, demonstrates superior performance in predicting drug-disease associations by leveraging both disease and drug features within a heterogeneous network. Its solid performance reveals its possibilities for therapeutic repurposing, therefore streamlining the drug research and development process [69].

Collectively, these studies underscore the efficacy of GNNs and their variants in modeling complex biomedical relationships for DDA prediction. While GCNs excel at capturing local neighborhood structures, incorporating attention mechanisms, as seen in GATs, allows models to evaluate the significance of several neighbors, enhancing predictive accuracy.

In order to predict synergistic medication combinations, Wang et al. introduced DeepDDS, a deep learning model that combines GNNs with attention processes.. By integrating drug molecular structures and gene expression profiles, DeepDDS achieved notable improvements in identifying effective drug combinations [70].

Wang et al. developed DTI-GAT, an end-to-end framework incorporating Graph Attention Networks (GATs) for drug-target interaction prediction. DTI-GAT assigns different attention weights to each node, facilitating the interpretation of the DTI topological structure and improving predictive performance [71].

Tanvir et al. proposed HAN-DDI, a novel model for the prediction of Drug-Drug Interaction using Heterogeneous Graph Attention Networks. Unlike traditional GNNs, their model applies attention to capture the varying importance of biomedical entities, improving interpretability and accuracy [72].

Huang et al. proposed HDGAT, a Hierarchical and Dynamic Graph Attention Network for the association prediction of drug-disease. Unlike traditional GNNs, HDGAT enhances representation learning using graph attention mechanisms at both layer and node levels, significantly improving predictive performance over existing models [73].

A Hybrid Transformer with Multi-level Fusion for multimodal knowledge graph completion was presented by Chen et al. Their innovative approach integrates visual and textual modalities through a hybrid transformer architecture, significantly improving the semantic depiction of entities and relationships. This fusion framework obtained cutting-edge performance in complex link prediction, entity alignment, and relation extraction tasks across multiple benchmark datasets [74].

.Table 2.2: Summary of Graph-Based Techniques for Predicting Drug-Disease Association

Method	Type	Key Features	Limitation
Hetionet [59]	Knowledge Graph-Based	Metapath-based reasoning; integration of 29 data sources	Requires manual feature engineering
COVID-KG [60]	Knowledge Graph-Based	Path ranking in COVID-specific KG	Specific to COVID-19 domain
KG-Predict [61]	Knowledge Graph-Based	Embeddings from heterogeneous sources	Relies on data quality
AMVL [62]	Multi-View KG Model	Fusion of CTPs, KG embeddings, LLMs	Computationally intensive
EDGAR [63]	Knowledge Graph-Based	Rule-based reasoning via enrichment	Complexity in rule mining
HGTDR [64]	Heterogeneous GNN	Hetero-graph transformer architecture	Transformer requires large data
CKG [65]	Causal KG	Formal causal inference with mediation	Needs curated causal knowledge
KGML-xDTD [66]	KG + ML Framework	Explainable treatment prediction via KG paths	Dependent on curated paths
Decagon	GCN	Multimodal graph; side effect prediction	Relational sparsity
GraphDPA [67]	GCN	Drug-pathway associations	Requires pathway graph construction
HINGRL [68]	Graph Representation Learning	Heterogeneous biomedical network	Complex integration
HEDDI-Net [69]	Heterogeneous Network Embedding	Drug and disease feature fusion	Scope limited to available data
DeepDDS [70]	GNN + Attention	Drug synergy prediction with gene expression	Data fusion challenges
DTI-GAT [71]	GAT	Attention-based DTI prediction	Scalability issues
HAN-DDI [72]	Heterogeneous GAT	Attention on diverse biomedical entities	High training complexity
HDGAT [73]	Hierarchical GAT	Multi-level graph attention	Model complexity

Hybrid Transformer [74]	Multimodal KG Completion	Visual and text integration	Requires aligned multimodal data
MMGL [75]	Multi-modal Graph Learning	Clinical and imaging data fusion	Generalization to other domains
HGNN-MCI [76]	Heterogeneous GNN	Fuses structural and functional brain connectivity	Requires neuroimaging data

Zheng et al. developed a Multi-modal Graph Learning (MMGL) System for predicting diseases. MMGL leverages adaptive graph learning to integrate multi-modal data, such as clinical and imaging information, capturing complex correlations between modalities. This end-to-end model improved disease prediction accuracy, demonstrating the efficacy of multi-modal fusion in biomedical applications [75].

Yin et al. presented a Heterogeneous GNN that fuses functional and structural connectivity for diagnosing mild cognitive impairment (MCI). By constructing homo- and hetero-meta-paths from rs-fMRI and DTI data, the model captures intricate brain connectivity patterns [76].

Despite advances, drug repurposing models face key challenges such as data incompleteness and noise in biomedical knowledge graphs, which hinder prediction reliability. Clinical adoption of deep learning models is challenging because they frequently lack biological interpretability.

Furthermore, generalizing predictions to rare diseases or novel drugs remains a significant hurdle. Looking ahead, integrating active learning can prioritize experimental validation more effectively, reducing lab effort. Additionally, cross-domain transfer learning leveraging omics data like genomics and proteomics holds promise for enhancing model robustness, especially in underrepresented disease contexts, supporting more accurate and biologically grounded repurposing outcomes.

2.4 Review on Cancer-Specific Target Discovery Using Multi-Omics Data

multi-omics data, including transcriptomics, metabolomics, proteomics, genomes, and epigenomics, offers a comprehensive and integrative understanding of cancer mechanisms by capturing diverse biological signals across multiple molecular layers, enabling precise characterization, prediction, and personalized therapeutic interventions. Each omics layer contributes unique insights; for instance, genomics reveals mutation landscapes, while transcriptomics provides gene expression patterns that are critical to tumor behavior.

Li et al. introduced CMLBS, a consensus ML-based signature to integrate multi-omics data for hepatocellular carcinoma (HCC) stratification. Their methodology combined ten clustering algorithms with 101 machine learning models, yielding two distinct molecular subtypes. Notably, one cluster demonstrated a significant survival advantage, underscoring the prognostic relevance of CMLBS. Furthermore, low-CMLBS patients exhibited superior immunotherapy responsiveness across independent cohorts, while high-CMLBS patients revealed differential drug sensitivity patterns, including heightened susceptibility to agents such as Alpelisib and Carmustine. These results illustrate the potential of CMLBS as a robust framework for precision medicine in HCC by guiding therapeutic decision-making [77]. Integration strategies can be broadly categorized into early (feature concatenation), intermediate (joint embedding or model-level fusion), and late-stage (ensemble prediction) approaches.

Tools like iCluster, SNF (Similarity Network Fusion), and MOFA have been widely employed for such tasks. More recently, Wang et al. proposed MOGONET, a novel deep multi-view framework that leverages GCN to integrate heterogeneous omics data for biomedical classification. The model is designed to jointly capture omics-specific representations while also learning cross-omics correlations, thereby aligning individual feature spaces with a shared decision-making process. MOGONET outperformed other cutting-edge integrative techniques in comprehensive assessments across several cancer datasets comprising DNA methylation, mRNA expression, and microRNA expression. Moreover, the framework was able to identify biologically relevant biomarkers, highlighting its potential not only in tumor classification but also in precision medicine applications [78].

Shoaib et al. utilized TCGA multi-omics datasets and demonstrated that joint embedding of expression, methylation, and copy number data enhances glioblastoma subtyping compared to single-omics approaches [79]. These integrative pipelines not only uncover subtype heterogeneity but also improve biomarker discovery and treatment stratification, especially in breast and colorectal cancers. The continuous evolution of integration tools and deep learning frameworks is transforming oncology into a truly data-driven domain. Traditional ML approaches like SVM, Random Forest, and LASSO regression have been applied to integrated multi-omics datasets, offering baseline predictive performance. However, these models often struggle with high-dimensionality and non-linear interactions inherent in omics data.

DL models have proven themselves in addressing these challenges. For example, Spooner et al. benchmarked ensemble ML techniques, including PB-MVBoost and AdaBoost with soft voting for multi-modal integration across cancer and IBD datasets. These ensemble methods outperformed early fusion techniques, improving both predictive accuracy and feature stability [80,81]. Wu and Fang proposed SAEsurv-net, a stacked autoencoder-based architecture tailored for cancer survival prediction. By employing a two-stage dimensionality reduction strategy, the model effectively mitigated the curse of dimensionality while simultaneously addressing the heterogeneity inherent in multi-omics datasets. The first stage of autoencoders focused on removing heterogeneities arising from differences in data types and sizes, while the second stage integrated the diverse omics features into a unified representation. This hierarchical design enabled the extraction of more informative and biologically meaningful features. Experimental evaluations on TCGA cancer cases demonstrated that SAEsurv-net outperformed single-omics methods, in addition to several cutting-edge integrative methods [81].

In a similar vein, Lin et al. presented DeepMO, a deep NN framework for categorizing breast cancer subtypes that integrates multi-omics data, such as DNA methylation, mRNA expression, and copy number variation (CNV).. Their study emphasized that the integration of heterogeneous omics data enhances the ability to capture intrinsic biological differences across cancer subtypes, thereby improving recognition accuracy. The proposed model employed an encoding subnetwork for feature representation and a classification subnetwork for subtype prediction, achieving superior performance compared to single-omics approaches and existing multi-omics methods. Furthermore, the study demonstrated the role of feature selection in refining predictive accuracy and provided biological insights through gene ontology and pathway enrichment analyses, underscoring the potential of DeepMO in advancing cancer subtype characterization [82]. Their model showed superior results in tasks with many classes as well as binary, validating the utility of feature selection. Moon and Lee introduced MOMA, a multi-task attention-based model that enhances interpretability and prediction by assigning pathway-level importance weights within the integrated omics landscape. The framework vectorizes features and biological modules through a geometric representation, enabling the model to capture critical processes across heterogeneous omics data. By incorporating an attention mechanism, MOMA prioritizes biologically meaningful modules that contribute significantly to diagnostic outcomes. Their experiments on Alzheimer's disease and various cancer datasets demonstrated not only superior predictive performance but also improved interpretability of results. Furthermore, comparative evaluations validated the effectiveness of attention integration in enhancing biological insight [83]. Despite their strengths, deep models often face shortcomings, including limited interpretability, susceptibility to overfitting, and poor generalizability across diverse cancer types.

Neuro-symbolic and explainable AI approaches are increasingly applied to biomedical research to bridge the gap between predictive performance and interpretability. These models combine the pattern recognition power of deep learning with rule-based reasoning or symbolic knowledge, enabling insights that are biologically meaningful.

Chatzianastasis et al. introduced an Explainable Multilayer Graph Neural Network (EMGNN) designed for cancer gene prediction, which combines multi-omics information with multilayer gene–gene interaction networks. The model demonstrated strong predictive performance and also provided molecular-level feature importance, making gene prioritization interpretable in the context of biological pathways [84].

Tripathy et al. proposed an explainable GNN framework that integrates identifying biomarkers among interacting domains using multi-omics data and prior biological knowledge. Their approach highlights biologically meaningful subgraphs and improves biomarker discovery while maintaining transparency of decision processes [85].

Baugh et al. analyzed the role of neuro-symbolic rule learning in addressing real-life classification challenges, emphasizing the extraction of symbolic rules from deep neural models. Although not cancer-specific, this work demonstrates how integrating symbolic reasoning enhances interpretability and provides a pathway for transparent biomedical decision-making [86]. Collectively, these approaches illustrate that hybrid models can improve trust in AI-driven biomarker discovery by offering interpretability through graph structures or rule extraction. However, their adoption in clinical pipelines is still challenged by data sparsity, noisy biological knowledge, and the computational overhead of symbolic reasoning.

Beyond MOGONET and DeepMO, foundational integrative frameworks established much of today's practice. Early joint latent-space models, such as iCluster co-modeled copy-number and expression to uncover clinically meaningful subtypes, setting the stage for multi-view representations in cancer cohorts [87]. By incorporating associations across heterogeneous data types within a unified latent variable framework, iCluster moved beyond ad hoc integration and enabled statistically robust subtype discovery. Its application to breast and lung cancer highlighted how weak but consistent cross-omics signals could be leveraged to reveal novel molecular subgroups, influencing the trajectory of integrative clustering approaches in precision oncology research.

Similarity Network Fusion (SNF) introduced a patient-similarity paradigm that builds per-omics graphs and fuses them into a consensus network; SNF consistently improved subtype resolution over single-omics baselines across TCGA-like settings, and remains a robust baseline for new graph-based methods [88]. By leveraging the complementarity of heterogeneous molecular layers such as miRNA profiles, DNA methylation, and mRNA expression, SNF demonstrated superior performance in identifying clinically relevant cancer subtypes compared to earlier integrative strategies. Moreover, its ability to enhance survival prediction underscored the clinical utility of fused similarity networks, influencing subsequent developments in network-based multi-omics integration.

Multi-Omics Factor Analysis (MOFA), a probabilistic framework for unsupervised integration of heterogeneous omics datasets, was first presented by Argelaguet et al. [89] . Latent factors that encompass both common and modality-specific causes of variation are inferred using MOFA, enabling systematic disentanglement of biological and technical heterogeneity across molecular layers. Applied to chronic lymphocytic leukaemia cohorts, it successfully identified clinically relevant subgroups and underappreciated drivers, such as oxidative stress response, while also supporting tasks like imputation and outlier detection. The framework further demonstrated utility in single-cell settings by uncovering coordinated transcriptional and epigenetic programs during cell differentiation, marking an important advance in multi-omics data integration.

Building upon this foundation, Argelaguet et al. extended the framework with MOFA+ [90], created to tackle the difficulties of integrating increasingly complex single-cell multi-modal datasets. MOFA+ employs scalable variational inference to efficiently reconstruct low-dimensional latent spaces while introducing flexible sparsity constraints that enable modeling of variation across both multiple omics layers and experimental groups. This advancement allows comprehensive integration of diverse cellular readouts, facilitating the discovery of coordinated regulatory programs at single-cell resolution. By enhancing scalability and flexibility, MOFA+ significantly broadened the applicability of factor-based integration approaches in modern single-cell multi-omics research. Factor models like MOFA and MOFA+ generalize PCA to multiple modalities, learning shared and modality-specific factors that capture biological and technical variation; their success in bulk and single-cell multi-omics has made factorization a standard for denoising, visualization, and downstream biomarker discovery.

In supervised integration, DIABLO (from the mixOmics suite) performs sparse, component-based fusion across modalities to maximize cross-omics correlation while discriminating phenotypes, yielding compact signatures that are easier to validate in the lab. More broadly, the mixOmics package provides a versatile framework for multivariate analysis, dimension reduction, and visualization tailored to heterogeneous omics datasets. By extending Projection to Latent Structures (PLS) models, mixOmics supports integrative analyses across multiple omics layers or even independent studies, enabling both unsupervised exploration and supervised classification. Its ability to identify molecular signatures in a holistic, systems-level manner has made it a widely adopted toolkit in integrative biology [91].

Complementing DIABLO's component approach, netDx frames integration as patient-similarity networks across omics and clinical features, then learns interpretable network combinations that highlight which data streams (e.g., methylation vs. CNV) drive predictions useful for communicating evidence in tumor boards. By leveraging similarity-based representations familiar to clinicians, netDx enhances trust and interpretability while maintaining strong predictive performance, outperforming conventional ML baselines in survival prediction of cancer. The framework handles missing data without imputation and supports pathway-level grouping of genes, offering mechanistic insights into predictive features. Through its Bioconductor implementation, netDx provides scalable workflows with built-in evaluation metrics and Cytoscape visualization [92].

Recent work also targets practical challenges like missing modalities and scarce labels. MAUI uses stacked autoencoders to derive "multi-omic fingerprints" that preserve biological signal even with modest sample sizes, aiding subtype discovery and outcome prediction. By integrating diverse molecular layers including genomic, proteomic, transcriptomic, and epigenomic data, MAUI captures complex, non-linear relationships across modalities. These learned fingerprints have been shown to accurately classify cancer types and subtypes while also associating with clinically relevant outcomes such as patient survival and therapeutic response. Importantly, MAUI supports interpretability by deconvolving latent features into subsets of genes and alterations with mechanistic relevance [93].

Likewise, miss-SNF extends the SNF paradigm to incomplete multi-omics, enabling integrative patient-similarity construction when some assays are absent, an everyday reality in real-world oncology cohorts. By adopting a multimodal message-passing approach, miss-SNF can recover missing patient similarities across networks, ensuring robust integration even when entire modalities are unavailable. This task-agnostic framework supports both unsupervised clustering and supervised prediction, achieving cutting-edge performance on TCGA datasets for subtype discovery, survival stratification, and outcome prediction. Importantly, benchmarked "amputation" experiments highlight that miss-SNF maintains predictive accuracy in cancer and Alzheimer's disease, demonstrating its practical utility for precision medicine under incomplete data conditions [94].

Autoencoder variants (e.g., contractive or denoising) further improve robustness and feature stability for subtyping and survival modeling under high-dimensional noise. Guo et al. [95] proposed a contractive autoencoder framework that constrains latent representations to be less sensitive to small perturbations, thereby enhancing feature reliability across heterogeneous omics modalities. By coupling this representation learning step with Cox proportional hazards regression, the model prioritizes survival-associated features, ensuring clinical relevance in downstream clustering. Applied to ten cancer datasets spanning four omics layers, the framework achieved better outcomes compared to current strategies, yielding greater concordance indices and more distinct survival stratification.

At the single-cell frontier, multi-omics assays (joint RNA-seq, ATAC-seq, methylation, and protein) expose cell-state programs and trajectory-level vulnerabilities that bulk profiles can mask. Reviews highlight analysis pipelines that borrow from bulk integrators (factor models, graph-based fusion, attention mechanisms) while accounting for sparsity and cell heterogeneity, enhancing target discovery by mapping pathway dysregulation at cell-type resolution. As summarized by Lee et al. [96], advances in isolation, barcoding, and sequencing technologies now allow for the simultaneous characterization of various molecular layers within single cells.

Table 2.3: Summary of Multi-Omics Cancer Target Discovery Methods

Method	Type	Key Features	Limitation
CMLBS Framework for HCC Subtyping [77]	Multi-omics Consensus Clustering + ML	Integrates 10 clustering algorithms and 101 ML combinations; identifies two HCC subtypes with survival and drug sensitivity associations.	May require large cohorts; computationally intensive; dependent on high-quality omics data.
MOGONET [78]	Graph Convolutional Network (Deep Learning)	Jointly learns omics-specific embeddings and cross-omics correlations for mRNA, miRNA, and DNA methylation.	Relies on graph quality; limited interpretability for clinical translation.
Integrative ML Approaches for Multi-Omics [79]	Traditional + ML Integration	Employs ML methods (RF, SVM, LASSO) and fusion strategies to combine genomics, transcriptomics, proteomics, metabolomics for biomarker discovery.	Susceptible to overfitting; limited handling of complex nonlinear interactions.
PB-MVBoost / Ensemble ML for Multi-Omics [80]	Ensemble Machine Learning (Late Fusion)	Compares boosted voting, meta-learner, and mixture-of-experts for multi-class clinical outcome prediction across omics modalities.	Performance depends on optimal hyperparameter tuning; interpretability remains challenging.
SAEsurv-net [81]	Stacked Autoencoder + Neural Network	Two-stage dimensionality reduction; stacked autoencoder integrates heterogeneous multi-omics data	Limited interpretability; requires large datasets
DeepMO [82]	Deep Neural Network (DNN)	Encodes mRNA, DNA methylation, and CNV data; separate encoder & classifier networks	Sensitive to feature selection; overfitting on small datasets
MOMA[83]	Multi-Task Attention Model	Vectorizes features; module-level attention for multi-omics integration	Requires extensive tuning; attention may overfit noisy modules
EMGNN (Explainable Multilayer GNN) [84]	GNN with multilayer integration	utilizes pan-cancer omics data and gene interaction networks, provides model-level and molecular-level	Requires multiple high-quality interaction networks; computationally

		interpretability via feature importance and gene set enrichment analysis	intensive for large-scale datasets
Explainable GNN for Multi-Omics [85]	Graph Neural Network + Set Transformer	Integrates multi-omics with biological knowledge graphs; provides biomarker interpretability	Dependent on knowledge graph quality; computationally expensive
Neuro-Symbolic Rule Learning [86]	Neural DNF + Symbolic Reasoning	Learns symbolic rules from deep neural features for multi-class classification	Limited biomedical focus; scalability challenged with large multi-omics
iCluster [87]	Joint Latent-Space Model	Co-models CNV and expression to uncover subtypes.	Restricted to linear relationships; limited scalability for high-dimensional modern data.
SNF (Similarity Network Fusion) [88]	Network-based Integration	Builds per-omics patient graphs and fuses into consensus.	Struggles with missing data; assumes homogeneous cohort size across omics.
MOFA / MOFA+ [89,90]	Factor Analysis (Probabilistic)	Learns shared & modality-specific latent factors; scalable inference in MOFA+.	Requires careful factor interpretation; sensitive to hyperparameter tuning.
DIABLO (mixOmics) [91]	Sparse Component-Based Integration	Maximizes cross-omics correlation while discriminating phenotypes.	May miss nonlinear interactions; requires balanced sample sizes.
netDx [92]	Patient-Similarity Network Classifier	Builds interpretable patient similarity networks with pathway-level grouping.	Limited scalability for extremely large cohorts; requires curated networks.
MAUI [93]	Deep Learning (Stacked Autoencoders)	Learns "multi-omic fingerprints" preserving biological signal.	Needs hyperparameter optimization; risk of overfitting in small datasets.
miss-SNF [94]	Network Fusion with Missing Data	Extends SNF to handle incomplete modalities via message passing.	Complexity increases with many missing modalities; performance sensitive to network construction.

Contractive Autoencoder Framework [95]	Deep Representation Learning	Learns robust latent features under perturbation, coupled with survival models.	Sensitive to training stability; requires careful regularization.
Single-cell Multi-omics Integration [96]	Multi-modal Single-Cell Analysis	Joint profiling of RNA, ATAC, methylation, protein; latent factor/graph-based fusion.	Data sparsity; high technical noise; costly assays.
DepMap (Cancer Dependency Map) [97]	Multi-omics + Functional Screens	Links CRISPR/RNAi gene essentiality with omics annotations.	Cell-line bias; may not fully capture tumor microenvironment.
LINCS L1000 (Connectivity Map) [98]	Perturbational Transcriptomics	>1M drug/gene perturbational profiles; reduced representation assay.	Reduced transcript coverage (inferred expression); lacks multi-omics layers.

Such integrative analyses reveal context-specific gene regulation and functional states, offering unprecedented insight into disease mechanisms and therapeutic targets. These advances dovetail with explainable GNNs and neuro-symbolic strategies to connect predictions to pathway-level or rule-level rationales vital for translational uptake.

Finally, resource ecosystems now close the loop from omics integration → hypothesis → target nomination. The Cancer Dependency Map (DepMap) integrates CRISPR/RNAi essentiality with multi-omics to chart context-specific gene dependencies and synthetic-lethal partners; recent "second-generation" maps couple large-panel screenings with multi-omic annotations and demonstrate translational target nomination across tumor types. Pacini et al. [97] extended this effort by profiling 930 cancer cell lines with rich multi-omic data and systematically linking molecular markers to genetic dependencies. By incorporating networks of protein-protein interactions and therapeutically relevant correlations, this framework prioritized 370 tractable anti-cancer targets, offering a clinically actionable roadmap for drug development.

In parallel, LINCS L1000 provides >1M perturbational expression profiles linking genes, drugs, and pathways, enabling signature-based drug repurposing and mechanism-of-action inference that can be aligned with tumor multi-omics to prioritize actionable therapies. Subramanian et al. [98] demonstrated that the reduced representation L1000 assay offers a scalable and cost-effective alternative to RNA sequencing, while retaining high reproducibility and broad transcriptome coverage through computational inference. This large-scale expansion of the Connectivity Map not only facilitates systematic exploration of drug-gene-disease relationships but also supports clinical translation by informing trial design, functional annotation of disease variants, and mechanism-driven therapeutic discovery.

Together with resources such as cBioPortal and TCGA-style repositories, integrative multi-omics platforms now enable end-to-end pipelines that span from data-driven modeling and interpretable ranking to preclinical validation of cancer-specific targets. The reviewed studies collectively underscore that multi-omics integration ranging from classical ML to advanced DL and attention-based frameworks, significantly enhances cancer subtype classification, survival prediction, and biomarker discovery. Importantly, the growing adoption of explainable graph-based and neuro-symbolic models, as explained by Chatzianastasis et. al, Tripathy et al., and Baugh et al., highlights a paradigm shift toward biologically interpretable AI. By bridging predictive performance with symbolic reasoning and graph learning, these approaches move beyond black-box outputs to provide traceable, mechanism-driven insights [84-86]. This trajectory establishes a promising foundation for explainable neuro-symbolic learning frameworks tailored to Drug-Target-Disease prediction across multiple cancer types, thereby advancing both interpretability and translational utility in precision oncology.

CHAPTER 3

DATASETS AND RESOURCES FOR THE PROPOSED METHODOLOGY

The effectiveness and generalizability of any data-driven research in drug discovery significantly depend on the quality, relevance, and diversity of datasets employed. This section gives a comprehensive summary of the datasets used to address the three core objectives of this study. Each objective demanded a distinct dataset strategy tailored to its specific goals and methodological requirements.

For the first objective, which focuses on predicting drug–target interactions (DTIs) using deep learning, well-established benchmark datasets widely adopted in the field were employed to ensure reproducibility and enable performance comparability with existing models. These datasets include curated DTI pairs along with affinity scores and drugs and protein representations.

The second objective, which involves drug repurposing through knowledge networks, required literature-derived datasets that encompass heterogeneous biological relationships among drugs, diseases, targets, and pathways. These datasets were extracted from high-quality biomedical knowledge bases and integrated to form a robust graph structure suitable for downstream learning tasks.

The third objective, which is concentrated on multi-omics-based prediction of therapeutic targets in cancer, resulted in the creation of a unique dataset, one of the key contributions of this research. Named OncoOmicsNet, this dataset was developed by aggregating and curating publicly available omics datasets (such as gene-expression and mutation profiles) from multiple open-source repositories and peer-reviewed literature. The collected data were carefully processed, normalized, and structured to make it directly applicable to deep learning models for precision oncology. This dataset fills a significant gap in the field by providing a clean, integrated, and task-specific resource tailored for multi-omics-based cancer target prediction.

The datasets used for each goal are described in depth in the sections that following, including their sources, structure, preprocessing steps, and relevance to the study.

3.1 Datasets for Drug-Target Interaction (DTI) Prediction

The KIBA dataset [99]and the Davis dataset [100] are two well-established datasets that are employed in the study to estimate the affinities of drug-target binding. These two datasets are both known in the fields of bioinformatics and cheminformatics as robust benchmarks, especially for the type of model that dispenses with explicit structure in the interest of numerical, sequence-based, or graph-derived representation. In these datasets, small molecules are described using SMILES (Simplified Molecular Input Line Entry System) strings, while protein targets are represented by their amino acid sequences. The interaction strength between targets and drugs is quantified through experimentally derived affinity scores (e.g., pKd values in the Davis dataset and KIBA scores in the KIBA dataset), which serve as ground truth labels for training and evaluating predictive models.

3.1.1 Davis dataset

The Davis dataset provides a subset of interaction data, having 68 small-molecule inhibitors and 442 human kinase proteins. The data set is from selectivity assays in which the experimental measurement of the interaction's strength is done using the dissociation constant (K_d), measured in nanomolar concentrations. K_d is inversely proportional to binding strength. Stronger values correspond to weaker interactions. The raw values are log-transformed to aid computational stability as well as interpretation. K_d values range continuously from 5.0 to 10.8. 30,056 known drug-target interaction pairs constitute the Davis dataset as a dense matrix suitable for model validation in early stages and performance benchmarking under fully characterized biological conditions.

Complementing the Davis dataset in scale and complexity, the KIBA dataset aggregates 2,116 small molecules and 229 protein targets, resulting in 118,254 experimentally confirmed DTI pairs after filtering. Unlike datasets reporting a single binding measure, KIBA integrates multiple assay types, Kd (dissociation constant, representing the equilibrium between bound and unbound states of a drug-target complex), Ki (inhibition constant, reflecting the concentration needed to inhibit half of the target activity), and IC50 (The concentration needed to cut biological activity by half is known as the half maximum inhibitory concentration). In practice, Kd values are often expressed as pKd (-log10Kd), where higher pKd values indicate stronger binding affinity. These heterogeneous biochemical measures are normalized and combined into a single quantitative metric known as the KIBA score. A lower KIBA score corresponds to stronger interaction strength between a target and drug, whereas higher values indicate weaker interactions. By abstracting diverse assay outputs into a uniform continuous scale, the KIBA score enhances comparability across different experimental protocols and provides a consistent foundation for benchmarking predictive models.

3.1.2 KIBA Dataset

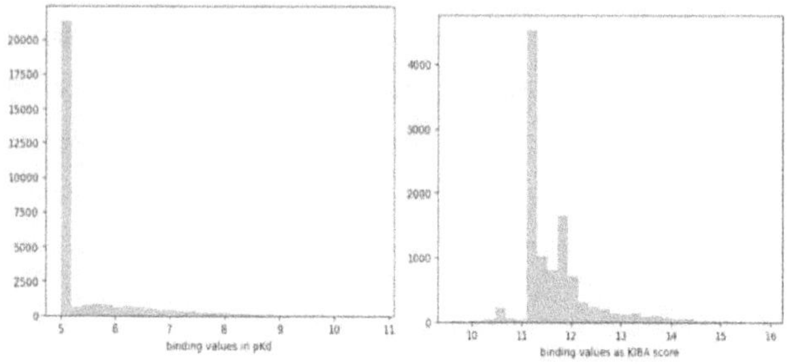

Figure 3.1: Binding affinity value distributions across the Davis and KIBA datasets

To ensure statistical robustness and minimize data sparsity, only drugs and proteins possessing a minimum of ten experimentally verified interactions were retained, aligning with methodologies established in previous benchmark studies. The KIBA scores span a range of 0.0 to 17.2, wherein lower values correspond to stronger binding affinities. Figure 3.1 and Table 3.1 depict the dataset's comprehensive statistical distribution and interaction landscape.

Table 3.1: The statistical information of the datasets

Dataset	No of drugs	No of proteins	Known DTI
Davis	68	442	30,056
Kiba	2,116	229	118,254

3.2 Datasets for Drug Repurposing using Knowledge Networks

In this study, the dataset utilized for drug repurposing through knowledge networks was derived from prior published literature, where significant efforts had already been made to integrate and curate relevant associations[101,102]. Specifically, a collection comprising 18,416 experimentally validated drug-disease associations was considered, involving 269 distinct drugs and 598 diseases. These associations trace back to entries within the

Comparative Toxicogenomics Database (CTD) [103], which served as a foundational source. The dataset, as employed in this research, is the result of a multi-stage aggregation and refinement process adopted from earlier studies, wherein diverse biomedical entities were structured into a form amenable to network-based computational analysis. This prepared dataset forms the backbone of the knowledge graph models applied in the subsequent analysis and is further elaborated in the following sections. These associations form the backbone of Drug-Disease Similarity Matrix, encoding each known therapeutic link as a binary or weighted edge that informs downstream graph learning.

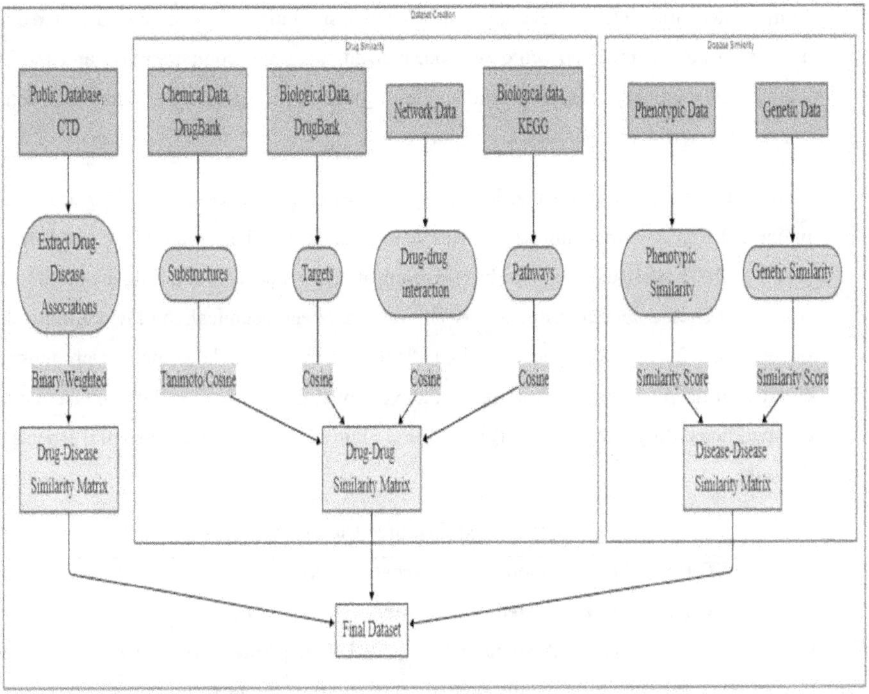

Figure 3.2 : Workflow for Multi-Source Dataset Creation

To capture inter-drug relationships, a comprehensive set of descriptors was derived from Drug Bank [104] and KEGG [105]. First, chemical substructures were abstracted into molecular fingerprints; pairwise Tanimoto and cosine similarities between these fingerprints quantify structural congruence. Second, drugs' target proteins were represented as binary vectors, with cosine similarity measuring shared biological targets. Third, interaction profiles derived from

DrugBank's drug-drug interaction network were encoded as adjacency vectors, with cosine similarity reflecting common interaction partners. Lastly, pathway co-membership from KEGG was converted into binary pathway indicators, compared via cosine similarity. These four modalities were subsequently fused through either simple averaging or a learned weighting function, yielding the final Drug-Drug Similarity Matrix that balances chemical, functional, and network-based affinities.

In parallel, disease entities were compared along phenotypic and genetic dimensions to construct the Disease-Disease Similarity Matrix. Phenotypic similarity scores were computed from curated clinical feature overlaps, while genetic similarity was assessed via shared disease-associated gene sets. Each score was normalized to ensure comparability, and the MeSH hierarchical ontology was employed to refine phenotypic groupings, reinforcing semantic consistency across related disease categories.

Finally, the three similarity matrices drug-disease, disease-disease, and drug-drug was co-integrated into a unified knowledge graph representation. This multi-view graph structure serves as the input to the proposed hybrid graph attention network, enabling the model to learn from explicit therapeutic associations as well as latent chemical, biological, and clinical patterns. By fusing heterogeneous biomedical data into a single graph, a rich substrate is created for deep learning algorithms to uncover novel drug-disease associations and advance computational drug repurposing. Table 3.2 and Figure 3.2 highlight the essential aspects of the datasets.

Table 3.2 : Multisource Dataset description

	Total Drugs	**Total Diseases**	**Documented Associations**	**Target Features**	**Enzyme Features**	**Drug-Drug Interactions**	**Biological Pathways**	**Chemical Substructures**
Main Dataset	269	598	18416	623	247	2086	465	881

3.2.1 Drug-Drug Similarity

The similarities between drugs are derived by analyzing their respective feature profiles, which are represented as binary vectors. In these vectors, each element corresponds to a specific characteristics such as a chemical substructure, biological attribute (e.g., enzymes or pathways), or network-based information like drug-drug interactions. The presence of the feature is indicated by a value of 1, while its absence is indicated by a value of 0. An 881-bit binary vector that reflects the existence of recognized substructures is used to represent each medication. Combined, these form a feature matrix used for computing drug similarity via various quantitative techniques.

Jaccard Index [106]: This method computes the proportion of shared features to the total distinct features between two drugs. Formally:

$$S^{d}_{ab} = \frac{F_a \cap F_b}{F_a \cup F_b} \tag{3.1}$$

Here, $F_a \cap F_b$, captures the shared elements in the feature representations of drugs a and b where $F_a \cup F_b$ refers to the union of all unique elements across their vectors

Cosine Similarity [107]: This metric calculates the cosine of the angle formed by two binary feature vectors., focusing on their directional alignment instead of their magnitude.

$$S^{d}_{ab} = \frac{F_a . F_b}{||F_a|| . ||F_b||} \tag{3.2}$$

$F_a . F_b$ denotes the inner product between the feature vectors corresponding to drugs a and b, while $||F_a|| . ||F_b||$ represent their respective Euclidean norms.

- **Euclidean Distance** [108]: It measures the direct spatial gap between two points represented in feature space:

$$S_{ab} = \sqrt{\sum_{n=1}^{N} \left(f_{a,n} - f_{b,n}\right)^2} \tag{3.3}$$

Let, $f_{a,n}$ and $f_{b,n}$ denote the value of the nth feature corresponding to drugs a and b, respectively, where N denotes the total number of features taken into account.

- **Manhattan Distance** [109]: This technique sums the absolute differences across all features:

$$S_{ab} = \sum_{n=1}^{N} \left|f_{a,n} - f_{b,n}\right| \tag{3.4}$$

The outcome of these computations is a drug similarity matrix S, where each cell S_{ab} represents the similarity score between drug a and drug b. Among these metrics, the Jaccard Index is especially advantageous for binary data, as it focuses solely on the presence or absence of features rather than their frequency or magnitude. This makes it particularly effective for capturing meaningful differences and similarities in drug properties.

3.2.2 Disease-Disease Similarity

To assess the semantic similarity between diseases and drugs in the dataset, the structural classification system of Medical Subject Headings (MeSH) [110] was utilized. MeSH provides a standardized vocabulary that organizes disease terms within a hierarchical framework using unique descriptors. Every disease is associated with a Directed Acyclic Graph (DAG) [111], which represents its position and relational pathways within the hierarchy.

Within this DAG, the nodes correspond to descriptors associated with disease A as well as all of its ancestral terms, while the edges represent the relationships linking each node to its ancestors. The DAG for a specific disease A is represented as:

$$DAG(A) = \left(V(A), L(A)\right) \tag{3.5}$$

Where:

- V(A) includes all the nodes, comprising disease A and its hierarchical predecessors.
- L(A) denotes the set of links between these nodes.

Each node v in the DAG plays a role in shaping the disease's semantic representation. The contribution $C_A(v)$ for a node is defined as:

$$C_A(v) = \begin{cases} 1 & \text{if } v = A \\ \beta \cdot \max\{C_A(v') \mid v' \in \text{ children of } v\} & \text{if } v \neq A \end{cases} \tag{3.6}$$

Here, the disease node itself (when v=A) contributes a value of 1. For ancestor nodes (v≠A), the contribution depends on the maximum contribution among its child nodes, scaled by a semantic weighting factor β, which in this work is set to 0.5, in accordance with standard methodologies. The semantic value of a disease A, represented as SV(A) is calculated by summing the contributions of all nodes present in its DAG. To assess how similar diseases A and B are semantically, the common nodes shared in their DAGs are considered. The similarity is computed as:

$$SV(A) = \sum_{v \in V(A)} C_A(v) \quad (3.7)$$

$$Sim_{A,B} = \frac{\sum_{v \in V(A) \cap V(B)} (C_A(v) + C_B(v))}{SV(A) + S\ (B)} \quad (3.8)$$

In the given formula, $V(A) \cap V(B)$ refers to the nodes that are mutual to both diseases A and B, and $C_A(v) + C_B(v)$ quantifies the combined influence of each mutual node on the semantic scores assigned to both diseases.

3.3 Datasets for Multi-Omics-Based Cancer Target Prediction

The creation of a comprehensive multi-omics dataset was a crucial step in developing the neuro-symbolic drug-target-disease prediction framework. This dataset integrated validated positive target genes, curated negative non-target genes, gene–gene interaction features, and multi-omics profiles, enabling robust and biologically informed learning across multiple cancer types. Figure 3.3 illustrates the complete workflow, encompassing data collection, preprocessing, feature integration, and generation of the final dataset optimized for model training, validation, and evaluation.

3.3.1 Positive Target Gene Set

The positive gene set was curated to represent cancer-type-specific therapeutic targets. Initially, FDA-approved anticancer drugs for each cancer type were retrieved from the National Cancer Institute (NCI) Drug Dictionary. For each drug, drug-gene interactions were obtained from the Drug-Gene Interaction Database (DGIdb) [112] and Cancer Gene Census (CGC) [113], ensuring that only validated or clinically supported gene targets were included. This step yielded the positive target set, which formed the basis of the proposed supervised learning framework.

To enrich this positive set, biomarker and cancer driver genes showing significant overexpression or clinical relevance were included. Expression statistics were derived from

The Cancer Genome Atlas (TCGA) [114], while mutation data were cross-checked with COSMIC [115]. Only genes with reviewed SwissProt records from UniProt [116] were retained to maintain the accuracy and biological validity of the positive target set.

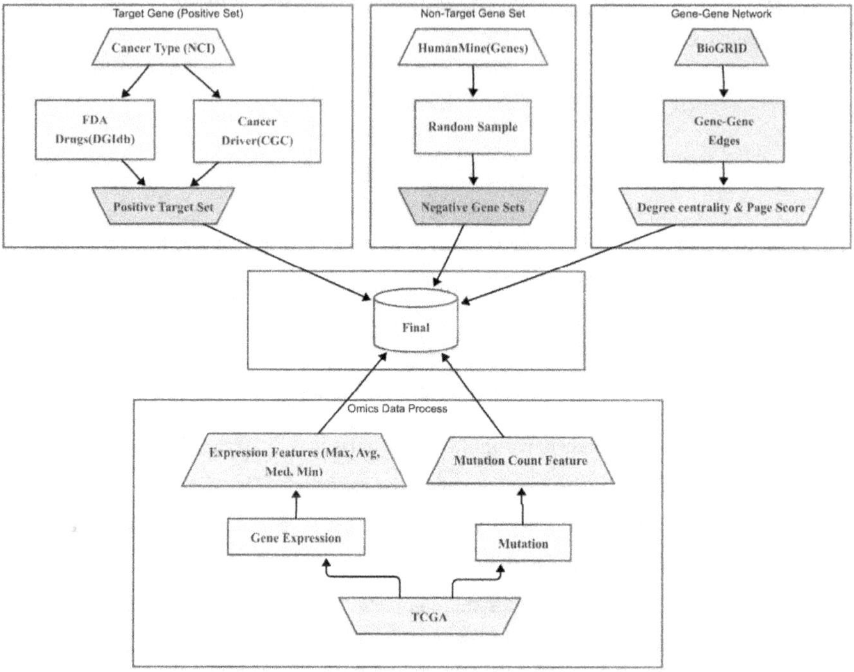

Figure 3.3 : Workflow of multi-omics Dataset Generation

3.3.2 Negative Gene Set

A negative set of non-target genes was constructed to create a balanced dataset for classification. First, the full list of human protein-coding genes was obtained from HumanMine, a repository integrating genomic and proteomic data. Genes already present in the positive target set were removed to avoid data leakage. Random sampling without replacement was then performed to select non-target genes. This balanced design is essential for machine learning tasks, as it mitigates the risk of bias toward the majority class and enhances predictive performance for minority (target) genes.

3.3.3 Gene-Gene Interaction Network Features

To incorporate biological network context, a gene-gene interaction network was constructed using BioGRID [117]. This database provides curated protein-protein interaction (PPI) edges, allowing us to represent the topological role of each gene in the cellular interaction landscape.

From this network, two fundamental graph-theoretic features were computed for each gene:

- Degree Centrality, which measures a gene's number of direct connections and identifies hub genes.
- PageRank Score, representing a gene's overall impact in the PPI network.

These features are particularly valuable for identifying potential oncogenic hubs and network-critical targets that could contribute to tumorigenesis or therapy response.

3.3.4 Multi-Omics Data Integration

The multi-omics component provides a rich feature space capturing gene-level molecular characteristics, adapted from prior published methodologies [118]. Omics data were retrieved from TCGA using the TCGAbiolinks package [119,120] , covering multiple cancer types. For each cancer type, a curated set of patient samples was identified using TCGA barcodes, and a corresponding gene list was established to extract relevant omics features, including gene expression profiles and mutation data. Gene expression data were extracted using the Illumina HiSeq platform, while mutation annotations were obtained via MAF files, indicating mutation presence per gene. Expression features were summarized across samples using statistical metrics maximum, average, median, and minimum while mutation features captured the count of gene-level alterations. All features underwent min-max normalization and were combined with curated positive and negative gene sets and network-derived centrality metrics. The resulting dataset integrates transcriptional, mutational, and network-level signals, forming a comprehensive foundation for predictive modeling and drug repurposing analysis.

CHAPTER 4
AN ENHANCED NEURAL NETWORK APPROACH FOR PREDICTING DRUG-TARGET INTERACTIONS

4.1 Introduction

In recent years, repurposing existing drugs has gained attention as a promising strategy within pharmaceutical science, offering a means to significantly lower both development time and financial investment compared to traditional drug discovery pipelines. This approach leverages previously approved compounds to explore alternative therapeutic applications, potentially bypassing early-stage clinical evaluations and expediting the overall process [121]. A central challenge in this domain involves reliably identifying interactions among biological targets of a drug, typically proteins, and the drug itself, referred to as DTIs. These associations plays a crucial part not only in uncovering new treatment possibilities but also in revealing adverse effects and underlying pharmacological mechanisms, which is especially valuable in the context of rapidly spreading diseases such as COVID-19 [122].

Experimental methods such as protein microarrays and affinity chromatography are traditionally used to validate DTIs. However, given the vast number of potential drug-protein combinations, these laboratory-based techniques are impractical for large-scale screening. They are resource-intensive, time-consuming, and often require specialized knowledge and infrastructure [123]. As a result, computational models have gained traction as efficient and scalable alternatives for predicting DTIs.

Conventional computational techniques for DTI prediction generally fall into three categories: text mining, biological feature-based models, and network-based approaches [124]. Text mining relies on descriptive data about drugs, while biological models use chemical and protein descriptors combined with classical ML algorithms such as Naive Bayes (NB), Random Forest (RF), SVM, and K-Nearest Neighbors (KNN) [125,126]. Although these models offer interpretability, they often require handcrafted features, struggle with high-dimensional data, and underperform in capturing complex nonlinear interactions. Moreover, they frequently assume balanced datasets, an assumption rarely met in real-world DTI scenarios, where known drug-target pairs (positive samples) are vastly outnumbered by unknown or non-interacting pairs (negative samples) [127–129].

DL models have been used more frequently for DTI prediction in order to get over these restrictions. These models eliminate the burden of manually engineering features via learning hierarchical data representations directly from raw sequences, such as amino acid sequences for proteins and SMILES strings for drugs. Architectures like Gated Recurrent Units (GRUs), CNNs, RNNs, and Long Short-Term Memory (LSTM) networks have shown substantial promise in extracting semantic, sequential, and structural features from these sequences [17,130,131].

However, despite their success, standalone CNNs or LSTMs face certain bottlenecks. CNNs are efficient in capturing localized patterns, but may fail to grasp long-range dependencies essential for capturing long-range interactions between protein residues and drug binding regions [132]. On the other hand, LSTMs are capable of modeling sequential data but can encounter vanishing gradient problems, especially when handling lengthy and complex input sequences. Furthermore, existing models often fail to effectively manage imbalanced datasets or exhibit poor generalization when exposed to noisy and sparse data, which is common in biochemical and pharmacological contexts [133,134].

To tackle the intertwined challenges of data imbalance and prediction inefficiency, this research introduces an automated, dual deep learning-based framework for robust DTI prediction. The proposed framework integrates two complementary approaches: (i) A binding affinity prediction model optimized using Honey Badger Optimization (HBO) for enhanced hyperparameter tuning in imbalanced settings and (ii) A binding affinity prediction model optimized using the Layer-wise Adaptive Moments (LAMB) optimizer for improved training efficiency and robust affinity estimation.

- Drug-Target Interaction (DTI) Identification using Honey Badger Optimization (HBO)

This approach employs a hybrid deep architecture that integrates 1D CNNs for local pattern detection, a Self-Attention-enhanced LSTM (SA-LSTM) for capturing long-range dependencies, and SMOTE with clustering to mitigate imbalance in training data. Honey Badger Optimization (HBO), a nature-inspired metaheuristic algorithm, is applied to optimize critical hyperparameters such as learning rate, dropout ratio, and layer dimensions, thereby improving robustness in high-dimensional and skewed datasets

- Drug-Target Binding Affinity Prediction using LAMB Optimizer

The second approach, termed FusionNet, combines CNNs, LSTMs, and Transformer layers to leverage both dependents both locally and globally in biological sequences.The self-attention mechanism of the Transformer allows the model to dynamically emphasize critical subsequences within drug or protein inputs. To ensure scalability and stable convergence on large biochemical datasets, the model incorporates the LAMB optimizer, which adaptively tunes learning rates at the layer level, improving both convergence speed and generalization under noisy conditions.

Together, these two affinity prediction strategies form a thorough approach that tackles the problems of imbalance and optimization in the prediction of drug-target binding affinity. The following sections of this thesis will explore related works, present detailed methodologies for each approach, and compare performance on benchmark datasets (Davis and KIBA) using industry-standard evaluation metrics.

4.2 Problem Formulation

In this study, both drug and protein data are represented as sequences to facilitate interaction prediction between them. The objective is to model and infer the relationships that may exist between a given drug sequence and a corresponding protein sequence. Each element in a numerical vector that represents a drug sequence represents a distinct structural or chemical characteristic of the molecule. As an example, a small-molecule compound represented using the SMILES notation

CC1=C2C=C(C=CC2=NN1)C3=CC(=CN=C3)OCC(CC4=CC=CC=C4)N

is transformed into a sequence of tokens or embeddings that preserve its molecular characteristics in vectorized form. Similarly, a protein sequence is converted into a fixed-length vector by mapping its amino acid sequence into a numerical representation. For instance, the protein sequence (eg. MKKFFDSRREQGGSGLGS). It is translated into a series of word-level or residue-level features that represent the biochemical properties of each amino acid. The combined representation, referred to as a Drug-Protein Pair (DPP) sequence, is constructed by concatenating both the encoded drug and protein sequences. In the given example, the DPP would be:

[CC1=C2C=C(C=CC2=NN1)C3=CC(=CN=C3)OCC(CC4=CC=CC=C4)N, MKKFFDSRREQGGSGLGS]

This paired input serves as the foundation for downstream interaction modelling, enabling the learning architecture to explore the joint feature space of molecular and protein-level information.

4.3 Methodology

4.3.1 Drug Target Affinity (DTA) Identification Using HBO-Based 1DCNN-SA-LSTM

In this study, a hybrid deep learning model 1DCNN-SA-LSTM-HBO is developed to predict drug-target affinities by considering both local and sequential features. The architecture combines 1D Convolutional Neural Networks (1DCNN) for extracting localized patterns from input sequences and a Self-Attention Long Short-Term Memory (SA-LSTM) module, enhanced through Honey Badger Optimization (HBO), to capture long-range dependencies effectively.

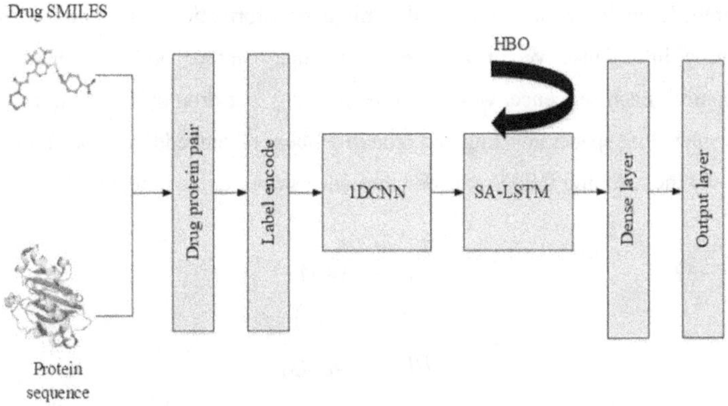

Figure 4.1: Structure of proposed HBO-based DTA model

As depicted in Figure 4.1, drug and protein sequences serve as the model's input, each of which is handled as a string of tokens or characters. These are first encoded using a Word2Vec embedding layer, which creates dense vector representations from the textual sequences that retain semantic and syntactic relationships.

Before model training, the issue of data imbalance is addressed using a SMOTE technique augmented with hierarchical clustering. This step ensures that synthetic samples are generated within biologically meaningful clusters, improving data diversity while preserving feature consistency. The encoded drug-protein pairs are then concatenated to form a joint input vector. The complete pipeline consists of several layers: an input layer, a Word2Vec embedding layer, a 1D convolutional layer for local feature extraction, an SA-LSTM module to model sequential dependencies, and finally, a dense output layer for prediction. Hyperparameters within the model are optimized using the HBO algorithm to maximize prediction accuracy and generalization across datasets.

4.3.1.1 Input Layer

The model accepts two distinct types of input sequences. The first represents the drug molecules using SMILES strings, while the second corresponds to protein sequences. Drug sequences are treated as character-based inputs, and protein sequences are handled as full strings. To convert these sequences into a format suitable for computational processing, label encoding is employed, transforming textual data into numerical representations.

4.3.1.2 Embedding Layer

The embedding layer functions as the initial transformation stage, converting raw input sequences into dense vector representations that capture both semantic and syntactic information. Each sequence, whether corresponding to a drug or a protein, is mapped into a word embedding space. For drug and protein sequences, embedding is performed at the word level, and the resulting DPP is encoded through a shared embedding matrix:

$$e_d = E(w_d) \tag{4.1}$$

$$e_p = E(w_p) \tag{4.2}$$

$$DPP = [e_d, e_p] \tag{4.3}$$

where e_d and e_p denote the embeddings of the protein sequences and drug, correspondingly. w_d and w_p are the tokenized input words, and E represents the embedding matrix. The dimensionality of these embeddings is defined by a pre-specified vector size. The embedding technique adopted in this work is Word2Vec, which is intended to record the semantic links between words (tokens) according to the sequence's surrounding context.

SMOTE with Clustering following the embedding stage, a SMOTE, a synthetic oversampling approach, was utilized to balance the dataset classes. To enhance the biological relevance and coherence of the synthetic samples, hierarchical clustering is first performed to partition the dataset into groups of similar drug-target pairs. These clusters are created using characteristics like the chemical properties of drugs and structural or sequence-based properties of proteins. Once clustering is complete, SMOTE is independently applied within each cluster to balance data distribution locally.

This localized application ensures that synthetic samples are generated only from structurally and functionally similar instances, thereby preserving intrinsic feature correlations, maintaining biological relevance, and preventing the introduction of implausible or overly generalized synthetic data points during model training.

4.3.1.3 1D-CNN Layer

During model training, the concatenated Drug-Protein Pair (DPP) sequence is fed into a 1D-CNN to extract meaningful semantic patterns. This network consists of multiple layers: input, fully connected (FC), pooling, convolution, and output layers. The convolutional layer applies several filters on the input from the layer before it., enabling it to capture and extract local patterns or features. The transformation can be mathematically expressed as:

$$h_i^l = f\left(\sum_j h_j^{l-1} * W_{ij}^l + b_i^l\right) \quad (4.4)$$

In this formulation, h_i^l represents the activation of the i-th neuron in layer l, W_{ij}^l denotes the filter kernel weights connecting neurons, b_i^l denotes the bias, f represents a non-linear activation function applied post-convolution. The Rectified Linear Unit (ReLU), which is represented as the model's activation function,

$$f(x) = \max(0, x) \quad (4.5)$$

Following convolution and activation, a pooling layer is applied to downsample the output, effectively minimizing the number of parameters along with computational overhead while preserving the most salient features. This operation is given by:

$$p_i^l = \text{pool}(h_i^l) \quad (4.6)$$

where p_i^l is the output of the pooling layer at the neuron i, and pool() denotes the downsampling operation (e.g., max pooling).

The (FC layer transforms the pooled features into a 1D feature vector. It aggregates data from previous layers and enables high-level reasoning. The FC transformation is defined as:

$$y_k = f\left(\sum_j w_{jk} \cdot x_j + b_k\right) \tag{4.7}$$

Where , f is an activation function, b_k is the bias value, w_{jk} is the weight connecting neurons j and k , x_j is the input from the neuron j and y_k is the output of the FC layer neuron k.

4.3.1.4 *SA-LSTM Layer*

A Self-Attention-enhanced Long Short-Term Memory (SA-LSTM) network was used to successfully represent long-range dependencies in sequential data. The input gate (i_t), forget gate (f_t), and output gate (o_t) are the three essential gates that define the LSTM architecture. The forget gate chooses which information from the input sequence should be filtered away. It is stated as :

$$f_t = \sigma\left(W_f \cdot [h_{t-1}, x_t] + b_f\right) \tag{4.8}$$

Here h_{t-1} denotes the hidden state from the preceding time step, x_t represents the current input,b_f and W_f and correspond to the bias of the forget gate and weight matrix, and σ refers to the sigmoid activation function.

The input gate controls which updated information should be added to the cell state:

$$i_t = \sigma(W_i \cdot [h_{t-1}, x_t] + b_i) \tag{4.9}$$

$$\tilde{C}_t = \tanh\,(W_C \cdot [h_{t-1}, x_t] + b_C) \tag{4.10}$$

where b_i, b_C and W_i, W_C are biases and weight matrices $\tilde{C}_t$ is the candidate state.

The cell state and output are updated as follows:

$$C_t = f_t * C_{t-1} + i_t * \tilde{C}_t \tag{4.11}$$

$$o_t = \sigma(W_o \cdot [h_{t-1}, x_t] + b_o) \tag{4.12}$$

$$h_t = o_t * \tanh\,(C_t) \tag{4.13}$$

where b_o and W_o, are the biases and weights for the output gate.

The self-attention module enhances the LSTM by dynamically assigning importance to various elements of the input sequence. It learns the relevance of each token using attention weights. The computation is as follows:

$$u_t = \tanh\left(W_w h_t + b_w\right) \tag{4.14}$$

$$\alpha_t = \frac{\exp\left(u_t^{\mathrm{T}} u_w\right)}{\sum_t \exp\left(u_t^{\mathrm{T}} u_w\right)} \tag{4.15}$$

$$s = \sum_t \alpha_t h_t \tag{4.16}$$

where u_t is the transformed hidden state, α_t is the attention weight, u_w is a context vector learned during training, s is the final sentence-level feature vector used for regression.

Here, α_t represents the normalized attention weight, while u_t represents the feature importance score at the time step t. The terms h_t and s correspond to the hidden state output and the resulting weighted context vector, respectively. The parameters W_w and u_w denotes the learnable weights, and b_w is the associated bias within the attention mechanism.

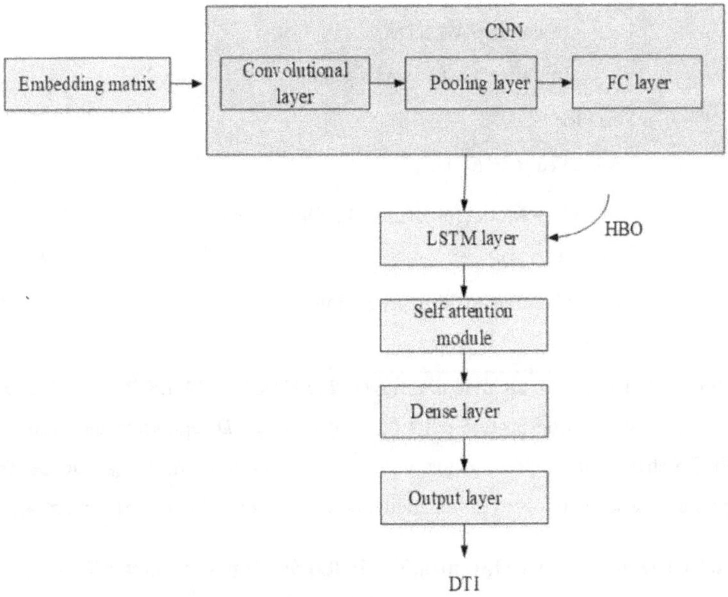

Figure 4.2 : The Structure of the proposed 1DCNN-SA-LSTM model

The resulting context vector produced by the self-attention-enhanced LSTM (SA-LSTM) is passed into a dense layer, which performs the final mapping required to calculate the Drug-Target Affinity (DTA) score. To ensure the prediction remains within limits, constraining the prediction at the output using a sigmoid activation function within the interval [0,1], aligning with the affinity score's normalized range.

Algorithm 4.1: 1DCNN-SA-LSTM

Input: $D - P$ sequences and actual binding affinity
Output: Binding affinity prediction
for every $D - P$ do
Input $D - P$
Compute embeddings as in Eq. 4.1 and Eq 4.2.
Concatenate embeddings as in Eq. 4.3
Create an Embedding matrix E_m
Initialize 1DCNN
Initialize SA-LSTM
Initialize $\mathrm{Re}LU$ and sigmoid
end for
Model (input E_m)
Model $\rightarrow$ Model (algorithm 4.2 Optimizer)
Predict $D - P$
return Binding affinity prediction
End

Figure 4.2 illustrates the architectural flow of the 1D-CNN-SA-LSTM model. The input to the model consists of drug-protein pairs ($D - P$), where D represents the drug encoded as a SMILES string and P represents the protein encoded as its amino acid sequence. The sequence of processing steps involved in this model is formally explained in Algorithm 4.1.

4.3.1.1 Honey Badger Optimization (HBO) for Hyperparameter Tuning

This work uses the Honey Badger Optimization (HBO) algorithm, a nature-inspired metaheuristic method to find the ideal hyperparameters for the SA-LSTM model, including the number of neurons, dropout rate, and LSTM unit size [135]. The optimization process proceeds through three main stages: population initialization, fitness evaluation, and optimal solution identification. The fitness function used to evaluate candidate solutions is defined as:

$$\text{Fitness} = f(x) \tag{4.17}$$

Algorithm 4.2: Pseudocode for optimizing parameters with HBO
Input: Initial hyperparameters for SA-LSTM, such as learning rate, number of LSTM units, and dropout rate Output: SA-LSTM configuration with optimal fitness value 1. Evaluate the fitness of each candidate xi using Eq 4.17 2. Identify and store the best-performing solution 3. While the termination condition is not met: a. Update δ using Eq 4.21 b. For each honey badger in the population: i. Compute intensity using Eq 4.20 ii. If a certain threshold is met, apply Eq 4.22 iii. Else, apply Eq 4.23 iv. Evaluate the new candidate's fitness. v. If new fitness is better, update the best solution 4. End While 5. Return the best solution (SA-LSTM with optimal parameters)

The HBO algorithm mimics the intelligent foraging behavior of honey badgers. To locate food sources, a honey badger relies on scent and guidance from a honeyguide bird. HBO models this behavior through two core operational phases: the honey-seeking phase and the digging phase. During the digging phase, the badger uses its olfactory cues to locate the prey. Upon reaching the site, it identifies the ideal spot to dig and capture the prey. The badger uses the honeyguide bird's help to find beehives during the honey phase.

HBO incorporates both exploitation and exploration to traverse the solution space effectively. The candidate population of potential solutions is expressed as:

$$X = \{x_1, x_2, \dots, x_n\}, x_i \in \mathbb{R}^d \tag{4.18}$$

Where x_i denotes an individual candidate in the population and d represents the dimensionality of each solution.

Initialization

The initial population is generated randomly within the defined upper and lower bounds:

$$x_i = L_b + r \cdot (U_b - L_b) \tag{4.19}$$

where $r \in [0,1]$ is a random scalar, and U_b and L_b are upper bounds and the lower and of the search space.

Describing Intensity

Intensity measures how strongly the prey emits a signal (analogous to fitness) and its distance from the honey badger. It influences the speed of movement; stronger signals lead to faster convergence.

$$I = r \cdot \frac{S}{D} \tag{4.20}$$

where D is the distance between the candidate and the target solution, r is a random number, and S represents the strength (fitness).

Updating Density

This introduces a time-dependent randomization factor that enables the algorithm to shift from exploration to exploitation over iterations:

$$\delta = \delta_0 \cdot \left(1 - \frac{t}{T_{\max}}\right) \tag{4.21}$$

where δ_0 denotes a constant, t corresponds to the current iteration number, and $T_{\max}$ refers to the maximum iterations allowed.

$$X = \{x_1, x_2, \dots, x_n\}, x_i \in \mathbb{R}^d \tag{4.22}$$

where x_i represents an individual candidate in the population and d is the dimensionality of each solution.

Digging Phase

In the digging phase, the honey badger executes a cardioid-shaped search movement to explore the local neighbourhood of potential solutions. The updated position of each candidate is computed as:

$$x_i^{new} = x_{prey} + F \cdot \delta \cdot r \cdot | 2 \cdot r - 1 | \cdot Flag \quad (4.23)$$

where $x_{prey}$is the prey (target) position, $F$is the search factor, $r$is a random coefficient, and *Flag* is a control parameter that alternates between exploration and exploitation modes to diversify the search behaviour.

Honey Phase

The honey badger locates the beehive (global best region) by following the honeyguide bird's guidance during the honey phase. The new position is updated as:

$$x_i^{new} = x_{prey} + F \cdot \delta \cdot r \cdot (x_{best} - x_i) \quad (4.24)$$

This stage emphasizes exploitation, allowing the algorithm to converge around the most promising candidate solutions.

Termination

The digging and honey phases are iteratively executed until the termination criterion (maximum iterations or convergence threshold) is satisfied. The best-performing candidate represents the optimal SA-LSTM configuration.

4.3.2 Drug Target Binding Affinity Prediction using LAMB optimizer for improved efficiency and stability.

Building on the strengths of modern DL architectures, this method presents a hybrid model that provides a strong framework for Drug-Target Binding Affinity (DTBA) prediction by combining CNNs, LSTMs, and Transformers. The model effectively captures hierarchical sequence features, local motifs, sequential dependencies, and long-range contextual interactions. The Layer-wise Adaptive Moments (LAMB) optimizer is used to guarantee effective and reliable training, particularly on large-scale biomedical datasets [136]. Designed for large-batch scenarios, LAMB adjusts learning rates per layer, enabling faster convergence and improved generalization. This integration enhances model scalability, stability, and accuracy in predicting drug-target interactions.

The suggested architecture, shown in Figure 4.3, uses a hybrid deep learning framework to extract local, sequential, and global contextual features from protein sequences and SMILES by combining 1D CNNs, Bidirectional Long Short-Term Memory (BiLSTM) layers, and Transformer blocks with multi-head self-attention.. To improve training scalability and stability, the LAMB (Layer-wise Adaptive Moments) optimizer is employed. An overview of the complete model workflow is presented as Algorithm 4.3a, 4.3b, and 4.3c. Output of Algorithm 4.3a is given as input to Algorithm 4.3b, and the output of Algorithm 4.3 b is given as input to Algorithm 4.3c

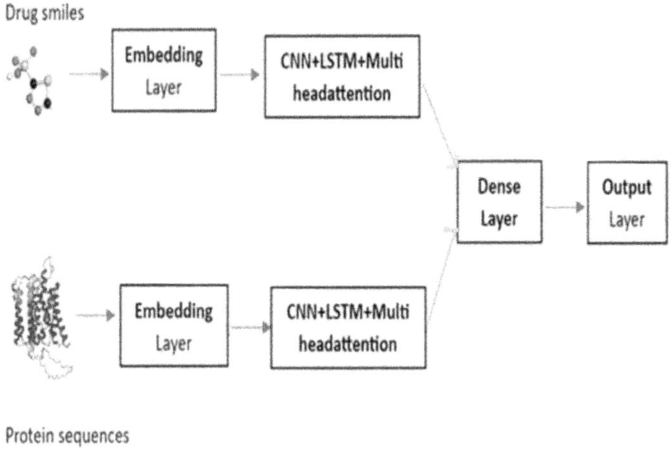

Figure 4.3: Structure of Proposed LAMB-based Model

4.3.2.1 Input Layer

The model accepts two parallel inputs: SMILES strings representing drug molecules and amino acid sequences representing proteins. These are pre-processed through character-level tokenization and padding to ensure uniform sequence lengths across the input space. The dataset is split into training and testing sets, after shuffling, and sequence representations are prepared for model ingestion.

4.3.2.2 *Convolutional Layer*

CNNs are applied to extract local structural patterns from both SMILES and protein inputs. Multiple 1D convolutional filters with kernel sizes of 4, 6, and 8 are used, selected through empirical evaluation to capture different subsequence motifs. The convolution operation for the ith the filter is formulated as:

$$f_i = x * k_i \tag{4.25}$$

Where k_i represents the convolution kernel of size i and x denotes the input sequence. Post convolution, max-pooling is utilised to down sample the output and retain dominant features:

$$p_i = \max(f_i) \tag{4.26}$$

The pooled feature maps from all filters are concatenated to form a unified representation.

Algorithm 4.3a: Drug-Protein Data Preprocessing and Sequence Encoding Framework
Input: Drug representations SMILES strings S, Protein sequences P, Interaction labels Y Output: $Padded_{\text{Smiles}}$ *and* $Padded_{Proteins}$ 1. Data Preparation 1.1 Randomize the order of samples in the dataset $D = \{(S, P, Y)\}$. 1.2 Partition the shuffled data into training and testing subsets: $\text{train\_smile, test\_smile} \leftarrow \text{S}$ $\text{train\_protein, test\_protein} \leftarrow \text{P}$ 2. Drug-Protein Sequence Encoding 2.1. Define a character-level encoding, $\text{Tokenizer}_{\text{SMILES}}$ 2.2. Apply the tokenizer to the SMILES strings used for training, $\{S_i\}_{\text{i}\in\text{D}}$ 2.3. Transform the SMILES strings into token sequences. $Seq_{\text{Smile}} = \text{Tokenizer}_{\text{SMILE}}\ (S)$ 2.4.Pad the strings to the longest possible length, L_{SMILES} $Paded_{\text{Smile}} = Pad(Seq_{\text{Smile}}, \text{L}_{\text{SMILE}})$ 2.5. Similarly, padding for proteins $Paded_{\text{Protein}} = Pad(Seq_{\text{Protein}}, \text{L}_{\text{Protein}})$

Algorithm 4.3b: Feature Extraction using CNN-LSTM Encoder
Input: $Paded_{\text{Smile}}$ *and* $Paded_{Protein}$ Output: Latent feature embeddings $H^{LSTM}_{\text{Smile}}, H^{LSTM}_{\text{Protein}}$ 1. Initialize two input layers, P_{input} for protein sequences and S_{input} for SMILES. 2. Use convolutional layers to encode SMILES and proteins, followed by LSTM layers. SMILE encoding: $E_{\text{Smile}} = \text{Embed}(\text{S}_{\text{input}})$ $C_{\text{Smile}} = Conv_{1D}\,(\text{E}_{\text{smile}})$ $H^{LSTM}_{Smile} = \text{LSTM}\,(\text{C}_{\text{Smile}})$ Protein encoding: $E_{Protein} = \text{Embed}(\text{P}_{\text{input}})$ $C_{Protein} = Conv_{1D}(\text{E}_{Protein})$ $H^{LSTM}_{Protein} = \text{LSTM}(\text{C}_{Protein})$

Algorithm 4.3c: Attention-Based Optimization and Prediction using LAMB
Input: Latent feature embeddings $H^{LSTM}_{\text{Smiles}}, H^{LSTM}_{\text{Protein}}$ Output: Predicted interaction scores Y' 1. Employ transformer blocks with LSTM layers and multi-head attention. For SMILES: $H^{Trans}_{Smiles} = \text{MultiHeadAttention}(H^{LSTM}_{Smiles})$ $H_{Smiles} = LayerNormalization(H^{LSTM}_{Smiles}, H^{Trans}_{Smiles})$ $F_{\text{Smiles}} = \text{LSTM}(\text{H}_{\text{smiles}})$ For Protein: $H^{Trans}_{Protein} = \text{MultiHeadAttention}(H^{LSTM}_{Protein})$ $H_{Protein} = LayerNormalization(H^{LSTM}_{Protein}, H^{Trans}_{Protein})$ $F_{Protein} = \text{LSTM}(\text{H}_{Protein})$ 2. Integrate the results of the protein encoders and SMILES. $F_{\text{combined}} = Concatenate(F_{\text{Smiles}}, \text{F}_{\text{Protein}})$ 3. Generate the interaction score as output, y'.

4.3.2.3 LSTM Layer

To capture sequential dependencies, the concatenated feature map is processed using a Bidirectional LSTM network. This architecture enables the model to gain knowledge from sequence contexts in the past and future. Let f be the input to the BiLSTM layer. The forward and backward passes are denoted as:

$$h = \mathrm{BiLSTM}_{\mathrm{forward}}(f) \oplus \mathrm{BiLSTM}_{\mathrm{backward}}(f) \tag{4.27}$$

where $\oplus$ indicates the concatenation of the hidden states from both directions.

4.3.2.4 Transformer Layer with Multi-Head Attention

Transformer layers are incorporated to improve the capacity to model long-range dependencies. A multi-head self-attention mechanism with 4 heads and key dimension of 64 is applied, where each head attends to different portions of the input.

The self-attention mechanism is calculated as:

$$\mathrm{Attn}\,(Q, K, V) = \mathrm{softmax}\left(\frac{QK^T}{\sqrt{d_k}}\right)V \tag{4.28}$$

Where, $d_k = 64$ represents the dimensionality of the keys and $Q, V,$ and K represents the query, value, and key, and matrices.

Following the attention operation, a feed-forward neural network is used to normalize the output:

$$H' = \mathrm{MultiHead}(H) \tag{4.29}$$

This sequence yields a final context-enhanced representation suitable for affinity prediction.

4.3.2.5 Layer-wise Adaptive Moments (LAMB) optimizer

To enhance model training, the LAMB (Layer-wise Adaptive Moments) optimizer was utilized, which is specifically designed to handle large-batch scenarios effectively. Unlike conventional optimization methods, LAMB dynamically adjusts the learning rate for each layer by considering both the norm of the layer's weights and the size of gradients. This mechanism promotes stable training behavior across deep architectures and facilitates faster convergence. Compared to optimizers like Adam, LAMB offers better scalability and efficiency, especially when training with large batch sizes (128 in this implementation). The learning rate was fine-tuned to strike a balance between stability and convergence speed. A dropout rate of 0.5 was also used to lessen the possibility of overfitting.

Mean Squared Error (MSE) was used as the evaluation metric to quantify the discrepancy between the predicted and actual binding affinity values and as the loss function during the model's 100 epochs of training..

4.4 Evaluation Metrics

In order to assess the performance of the proposed model, various commonly recognized regression metrics were used. These include Regression Toward the Mean (rm^2), Root Mean Squared Error (RMSE), Concordance Index (CI), and Mean Squared Error (MSE), . Each metric captures a different aspect of model behavior, from accuracy to ranking ability.

Mean Squared Error (MSE): The average of the squared deviations between the true values (y) and the anticipated values (ŷ) is known as the Mean Squared Error (MSE). It can be expressed mathematically as

$$\text{MSE} = \frac{1}{n}\sum_{i=1}^{n} (\hat{y}_i - y_i)^2 \tag{4.30}$$

where the number of samples is represented by n.. A smaller MSE value reflects higher accuracy of the model.

Root Mean Squared Error (RMSE): The square root of the average of the squared discrepancies between expected and actual values is known as RMSE. It is defined as:

$$\text{RMSE} = \sqrt{\frac{1}{n}\sum_{i=1}^{n} (\hat{y}_i - y_i)^2} \tag{4.31}$$

This metric is more interpretable because it offers error in the same unit as the output variable.

Regression Toward the Mean (rm^2): The rm^2 metric extends the squared correlation coefficient to evaluate how well predicted affinities align with observed values in regression tasks. It is computed using:

$$rm^2 = r^2 \times \left(1 - \sqrt{r^2 - r_0^2}\right) \tag{4.32}$$

Here, r^2 is the coefficient of determination (standard squared correlation), and r_0^2 is the squared correlation coefficient when the regression is forced through the origin (zero intercept).

Concordance Index (CI): CI evaluates the model's ability to preserve the ranking order of predicted affinities. It is particularly suitable for regression problems where the order of predicted values matters more than the exact values. CI is given by:

$$CI = \frac{1}{Z}\sum_{\delta_i > \delta_j} h(f_i - f_j) \tag{4.33}$$

In this equation, f_i and f_j are the predicted scores for samples with higher and lower actual binding affinities, respectively, Z is a normalization factor, and $h(x)$ is a step function that returns 1 if $x > 0$,0.5 if $x = 0$, and 0 if $x < 0$.

4.5 Results obtained by the proposed DTA

The results presented in this section are derived from the deployment of the proposed DTA model using the benchmark KIBA and Davis datasets, as compiled and described in Chapter 3 (Section 3.1).

4.5.1 Results obtained by the proposed HBO-based model

The subsequent section presents the evaluation results of the proposed model, including the accuracy-loss curves, precision-recall (PR) curves, and binding affinity matrices.

Figure 4.4 illustrates the accuracy and loss trends for the 1DCNN-SA-LSTM-HBO model on both the Davis and KIBA datasets. This analysis helps assess the model's convergence behavior and stability. Figures 4.4(a) and (b) display the validation and training accuracy and loss curves for the Davis dataset, while Figures 4.4(c) and 4.4(d) show the same for the KIBA dataset. It is evident that accuracy improves notably after epoch 25 and stabilizes around epoch 40. Correspondingly, the loss declines after epoch 25 and plateaus beyond epoch 40, confirming that the model avoids both underfitting and overfitting. Figure 4.5 shows the PR curve performance of the proposed 1DCNN-SA-LSTM-HBO model for the Davis and KIBA datasets. The area under the PR curve (AUPR) is used to evaluate performance under class imbalance conditions and assess the model's binary classification capabilities. For an ideal

DTA prediction model, the AUPR value should approach 1. From Figures 4.5(a) and (b), the model achieves AUPR scores of 0.9137 on the Davis dataset and 0.9156 on the KIBA dataset. The elevated PR curves reflect strong performance in terms of both precision and recall. This effectiveness can be attributed to the integrated use of 1DCNN, self-attention, LSTM, and HBO optimization in modeling complex drug-target relationships.

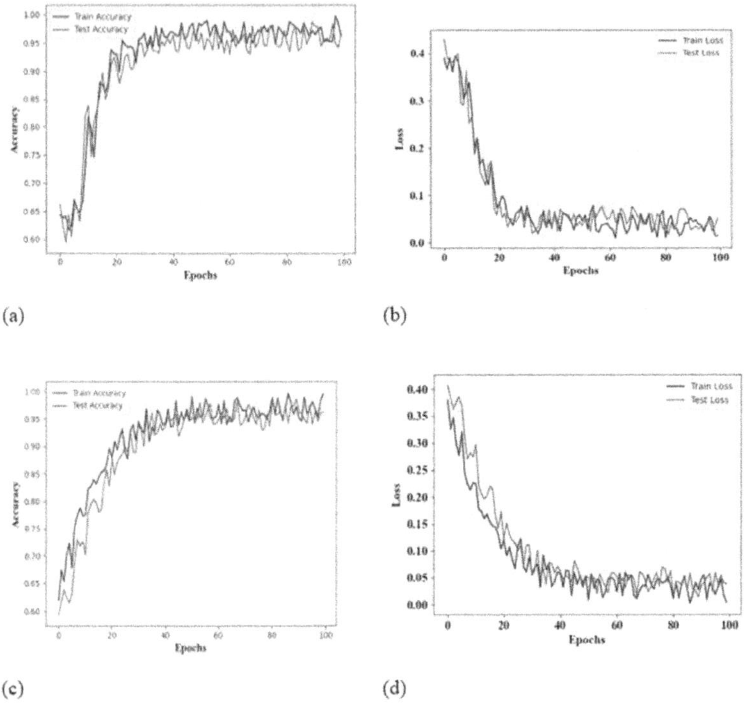

Figure 4.4: Accuracy–loss curves of the 1DCNN–SA–LSTM–HBO model on Davis (a, b) and KIBA (c, d) datasets.

Figure 4.6 presents the binding affinity plots for the Davis and KIBA datasets using the proposed model. In these plots, predicted values (blue dots) are compared against actual values (red line). A strong alignment between predictions and the reference line indicates better prediction performance. Figures 4.6(a) and 4.6(b) show that both datasets display high point densities around the red line. The Mean Squared Error (MSE) recorded for Davis is 0.2252, and for KIBA, it is 0.1058, demonstrating the model's strong predictive capabilities.

4.5.2 Results obtained by the proposed LAMB-based model

Across the KIBA and Davis datasets, the FusionNet model performs well in predicting drug-target interactions. With comparable validation values of 0.1852 and training loss and MSE of 0.1874 for the KIBA dataset, it demonstrated strong generalization and low overfitting risk.

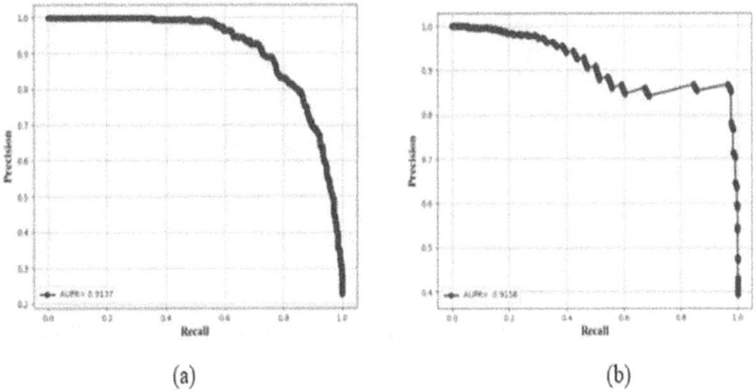

Figure 4.5: Precision–Recall (PR) curves of the 1DCNN–SA–LSTM–HBO model for Davis (a) and KIBA (b) datasets.

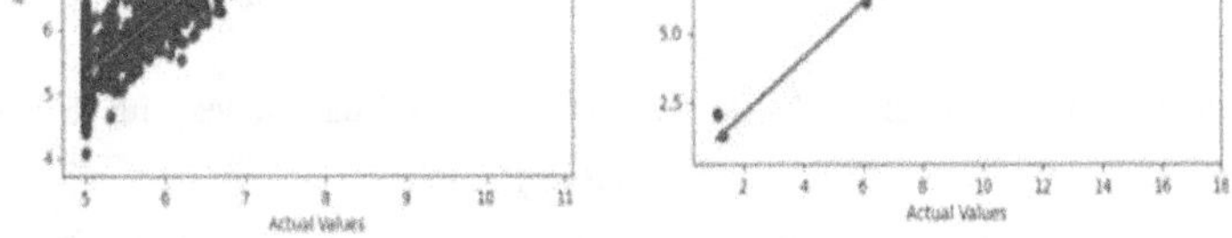

Figure 4.6: Affinity plots of the 1DCNN–SA–LSTM–HBO model for Davis (a) and KIBA (b) datasets.

For the Davis dataset, the MSE and training loss were recorded at 0.2073, and the validation metrics were slightly higher at 0.2296, indicating marginal variation yet retaining good predictive performance. The model's performance, depicted in Figure 4.7, tracks MSE over

100 training epochs. A steep decline in training MSE during the initial 10 epochs and the stabilization of validation MSE suggest efficient learning and strong generalization.

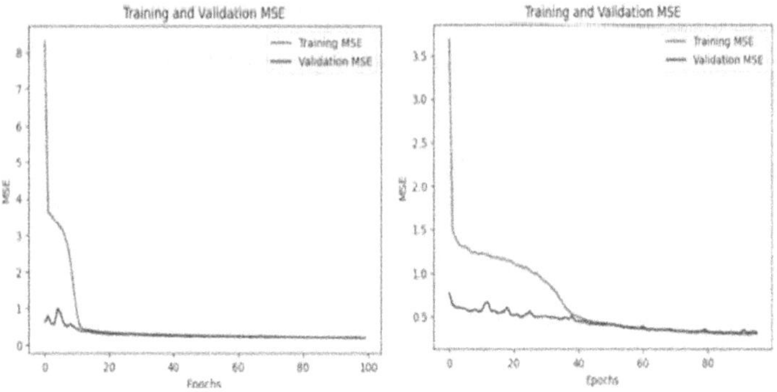

Figure 4.7: Training–validation MSE performance on Davis and KIBA datasets

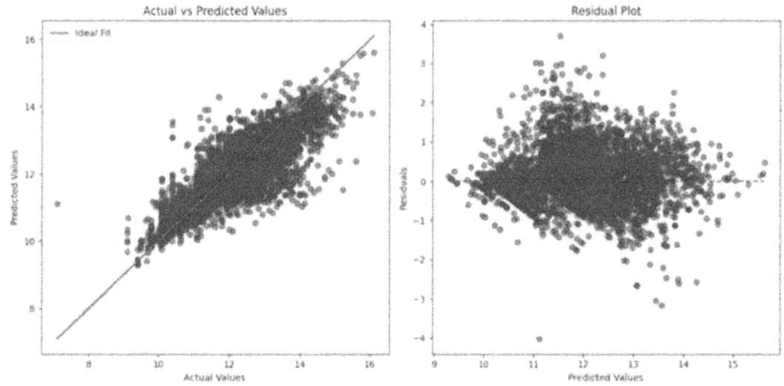

Figure 4.8: Evaluation of Model Predictions Against Actual Values with Residual Plots on the KIBA Dataset

Figure 4.9 presents "Actual vs. Predicted Values" along with residual plots for Davis dataset. For the Davis dataset, predicted values display wider dispersion, and residuals reveal pockets of prediction error. In contrast, as in Figure 4.8, the KIBA dataset results show tighter clustering around actual values, with residuals evenly spread around zero, indicating superior accuracy.

The KIBA dataset achieved an R-squared value of 0.710, demonstrating that 71% of the variability in actual values is accounted for by the model, signifying high predictive strength as in Figure 4.10. The Davis dataset produced an R-squared of 0.681, reflecting a slightly weaker correlation and reduced accuracy. Figure 4.11 illustrates an AUC of 0.90 for the Davis dataset, signifying excellent model capability in balancing sensitivity and specificity.

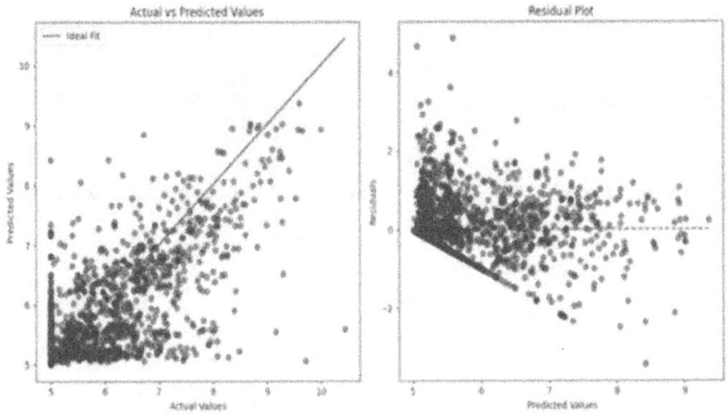

Figure 4.9: Evaluation of Model Predictions Against Actual Values with Residual Plots on the Davis Dataset

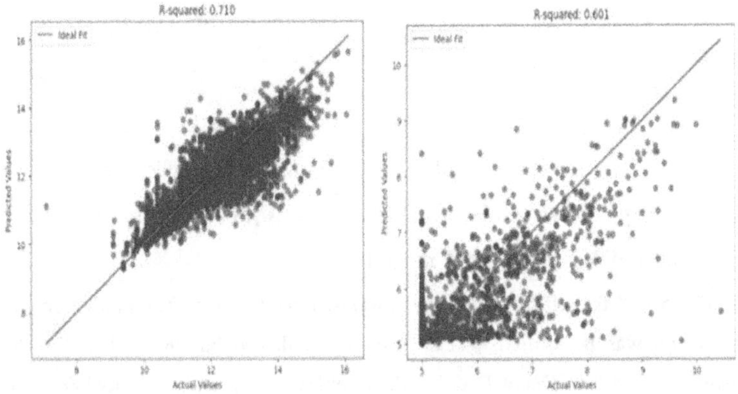

Figure 4.10: Evaluation of Actual vs. Predicted Values for KIBA and Davis dataset

Figure 4.12 shows a slightly higher AUC of 0.91, indicating marginally better performance. The results indicate that both models outperform random prediction, as denoted by the red dashed baseline.

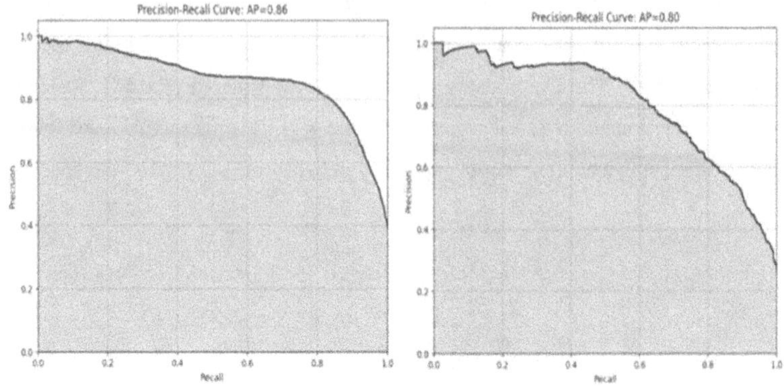

Figure 4.11: Precision–Recall–based evaluation of the proposed model across the KIBA and Davis datasets.

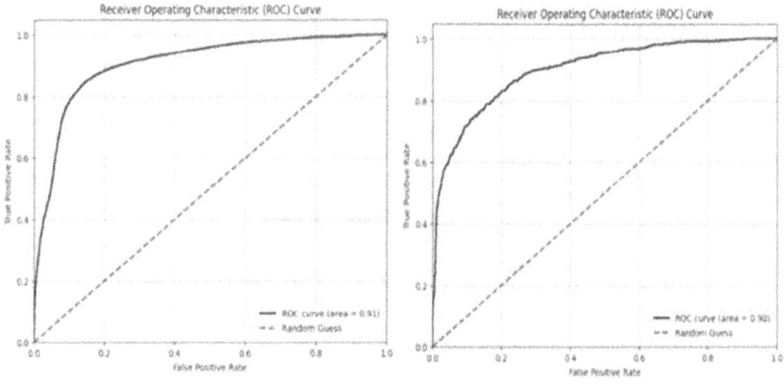

Figure 4.12: ROC curve for KIBA and Davis dataset

4.5.3 Comparative study of existing techniques with the proposed LAMB and HBO-integrated model

To determine the efficiency of the proposed models for DTI prediction, a comparative evaluation was performed against several established baselines, including SimBoost[50], GANsDTA [127], DeepCDA [128], DeepDTA[15], and Affinity2Vec[17], using two benchmark datasets: Davis and KIBA, as in Table 4.1. The models developed in this study, FusionNet (optimized using the LAMB optimizer) and 1DCNN-SA-LSTM-HBO (optimized using the Honey Badger Optimization algorithm), demonstrate substantial performance gains across all key metrics.

Table 4.1: Comparative Analysis of Existing Approaches vs. Proposed LAMB and HBO Model

Datasets	Methods	MSE	RMSE	CI	AUPR	rm2
Davis	SimBoost[50]	0.28	-	0.83	0.70	0.644
	GANsDTA [127]	0.27	-	0.70	0.69	0.653
	DeepCDA [128]	0.24	-	0.89	0.73	0.649
	DeepDTA [15]	0.26	-	0.87	0.71	0.67
	Affinity2Vec [17]	0.24	-	0.88	0.73	0.69
	Proposed (1DCNN-SA-LSTM-HBO)	0.20	0.45	0.96	0.9137	0.71
	Proposed (FusionNet)	0.20	0.55	0.89	0.86	0.681
KIBA	SimBoost[50]	0.22	-	0.83	0.76	0.629
	GANsDTA [127]	0.22	-	0.86	0.75	0.675
	DeepCDA [128]	0.17	-	0.88	0.81	0.682
	DeepDTA [15]	0.19	-	0.86	0.788	0.673
	Affinity2Vec [17]	0.12	-	0.91	0.91	0.765
	Proposed (1DCNN-SA-LSTM-HBO)	0.10	0.32	0.95	0.91	0.848
	Proposed (FusionNet)	0.18	0.40	0.88	0.81	0.71

On the Davis dataset, both proposed models achieved an impressive Mean Squared Error (MSE) of 0.20, surpassing prior methods such as DeepCDA (0.24), SimBoost (0.28), and

GANsDTA (0.27). The 1DCNN-SA-LSTM-HBO model further distinguished itself with a Root Mean Squared Error (RMSE) of 0.45 and a Concordance Index (CI) of 0.96, the highest among all models. It also reached a Precision-Recall AUC (AUPR) of 0.9137 and an rm^2 value of 0.71, demonstrating robust predictive accuracy and reduced bias. The FusionNet model, while slightly behind the HBO-based variant in CI and AUPR, maintained competitive scores (CI: 0.89, AUPR: 0.86) and outperformed all traditional models, validating the impact of LAMB optimization in stabilizing training and improving generalization.

On the more complex KIBA dataset, the HBO-optimized model again set a new performance benchmark. It achieved the lowest MSE (0.10) and highest CI (0.95), as well as a RMSE of 0.32, indicating its capability to make highly precise and consistent predictions. Notably, it also recorded an rm^2 score of 0.848, suggesting superior resistance to prediction bias and strong alignment with actual drug-target binding affinities. While the FusionNet model recorded a slightly higher MSE (0.18), it still outperformed DeepDTA, DeepCDA, and SimBoost, showcasing its utility in high-dimensional biomedical prediction tasks. In summary, the HBO-based 1DCNN-SA-LSTM model consistently outperforms existing methods, especially in settings with data imbalance and high interaction complexity, making it highly suitable for practical drug discovery pipelines. The LAMB-based FusionNet, although slightly less accurate, presents a highly stable and modular alternative with excellent performance, particularly in general-purpose DTI modeling scenarios.

Notably, both models diverge from traditional approaches by leveraging dynamic feature learning and optimization strategies, enabling them to generalize better across diverse drug-target pairs. The improvements demonstrated in CI, AUPR, and rm^2 confirm their utility in enhancing DTA prediction pipelines.

4.6 Conclusion

This research presented two innovative deep learning architectures for DTA prediction: 1DCNN-SA-LSTM-HBO and FusionNet-LAMB, each offering unique strengths in tackling the challenges of binding affinity estimation. The 1DCNN-SA-LSTM-HBO model demonstrated superior predictive capability by leveraging convolutional feature extraction, attention-based relevance weighting, temporal modeling through LSTM, and optimization via HBO. This combination significantly improved accuracy and generalization on benchmark datasets, achieving a CI of 0.96 (Davis) and 0.91 (KIBA).

Meanwhile, FusionNet, incorporating CNN, LSTM, and transformer layers, effectively modeled both local and global sequence characteristics. With the support of the LAMB optimizer, it maintained high stability and performance on large datasets, achieving MSE scores of 0.20 (Davis) and 0.18 (KIBA), with corresponding rm^2 values of 0.681 and 0.71, outperforming several leading models including DeepDTA, SimBoost, and GANsDTA.

Together, these models offer powerful and complementary strategies for DTA prediction. While HBO-based optimization excels in fine-tuning model parameters to improve generalization, LAMB-based optimization brings scalability and stability, particularly valuable for complex, large-scale datasets.

For future work, extending these frameworks by exploring advanced LSTM variants, more efficient metaheuristic optimizers, or integrating multi-modal data, such as 3D structural or genomic features, could further enhance prediction accuracy and biological insight. Moreover, incorporating unlabeled molecular data to learn unsupervised semantic representations and improving interpretability (e.g., linking attention weights to functional molecular subregions) could create new opportunities for comprehending drug-target mechanisms and quickening the medication development process.

CHAPTER 5
HYBRID GRAPH-BASED FRAMEWORK FOR DRUG REPURPOSING IN RARE DISEASES

5.1 Introduction

The preceding chapters established the role of deep learning in identifying drug-target binding affinities, demonstrating how molecular interaction modelling can aid early-stage drug discovery. However, narrowing down candidate compounds solely based on protein binding affinity offers a limited perspective, particularly when addressing real-world therapeutic challenges where multiple biological factors interact in complex, often nonlinear ways, including disease pathways, pharmacokinetics, and clinical phenotypes. To complement this protein-centric perspective and expand the practical applications of computational drug discovery, an in-depth analysis of drug repurposing is presented in this chapter, specifically through drug-disease association prediction.

Drug repurposing has gained considerable focus in recent years as a resource-efficient method for identifying alternative indications for existing pharmaceuticals. Unlike de novo drug development, with timelines exceeding a decade and requiring substantial financial resources, repurposing builds on known safety profiles, pharmacodynamics, and manufacturing protocols, substantially reducing the risk of clinical failure. This paradigm is particularly impactful in rare diseases, where small patient populations often disincentivize traditional pharmaceutical investment, leaving significant therapeutic gaps unaddressed.

Despite its promise, computational drug repurposing presents unique methodological challenges. Traditional machine learning models, while effective in some scenarios, often fall short in capturing the higher-order relationships between drugs and diseases, especially when these associations are not linear or explicitly labeled. Moreover, existing frameworks frequently rely on binary classification schemes, reducing the complexity of drug-disease interactions to a simplistic presence or absence decision. These models often ignore pharmacological nuance, such as dosage effects or pathway cross-talk, limiting their translational value. To overcome these limitations, this chapter introduces a Dynamic Heterogeneous Attention-based Drug-Repurposing Model (Dyna-HeteroAttnDR Model) designed for predicting drug-disease associations. This model addresses the aforementioned challenges by leveraging the expressive power of graph neural networks (GNNs) combined with hierarchical attention layers to enable finer-grained learning of node-level and topological features. Unlike previous approaches that focus solely on either local feature aggregation or global graph topology, Dyna-HeteroAttnDR balances both aspects through a multi-layer design incorporating sparse and dense convolutional layers, residual pathways, and layer normalization techniques.

The proposed framework begins by constructing a heterogeneous bipartite graph, in which nodes signify drugs and diseases, whereas the edges denote known or inferred associations. Similarity matrices between drugs and between diseases are utilized to enhance the network with contextual relationships, allowing the model to reason over indirect links and latent paths in the graph. This heterogeneity enables the learning model to integrate multimodal biomedical data while maintaining interpretability a critical aspect when considering clinical translation.

One of the key innovations of this work is the implementation of a hierarchical attention mechanism. At the micro level, attention coefficients are computed at the node-neighbor level to evaluate the significance of each local interaction. At the macro level, attention is extended across layers to dynamically weigh the contribution of various feature channels as the network deepens. These mechanisms collectively allow the model to identify and prioritize biologically meaningful patterns across the graph structure, improving not only classification performance but also model explainability.

Optimization of the Dyna-HeteroAttnDR architecture is achieved using Optuna, a robust hyperparameter search framework. Through a systematic exploration of parameter spaces, including embedding dimensionality, learning rate, dropout ratios, and layer configurations, Optuna identifies optimal settings that balance training stability with generalization performance. To further enhance model robustness, multiple attention weight initialization strategies, including Layer Prioritization, Uniform Allocation, and Dynamic Attention Weights, were investigated. Empirical results show that Dynamic Attention Weights, in particular, contribute significantly to learning expressive and diverse feature embeddings. Importantly, the proposed model is evaluated not just in general drug repurposing scenarios but also in the context of rare diseases, a critical area where conventional drug development timelines are often misaligned with patient urgency. Conditions such as Churg-Strauss

Syndrome, glioblastoma, cystic fibrosis, and Burkitt lymphoma present unique biological and therapeutic challenges that are rarely addressed by traditional pharmacological pipelines. The application of Dyna-HeteroAttnDR to these diseases not only showcases the real-world applicability of the model but also underlines its potential for translational impact in personalized and precision medicine.

While previous chapters focused on identifying high-affinity drug-target interactions using sequence-based learning and optimized deep architectures, this chapter complements that work by reframing drug discovery through the lens of disease biology. Here, the objective is not just to find molecules that bind strongly to proteins, but to uncover latent therapeutic relationships between compounds and disease phenotypes using graph-based modeling. By connecting molecular pharmacology with disease-level pathophysiology, the Dyna-HeteroAttnDR framework paves the way for an integrated, systems-level approach to drug discovery. The contributions of this chapter can be summarized in three parts,

- Presents a novel graph attention model capable of learning robust representations from sparse, heterogeneous biomedical data.
- Demonstrates the integration of adaptive learning techniques, including dynamic attention and Optuna-based optimization, to refine model architecture and enhance performance.
- Validates the model in the underexplored domain of rare diseases, showing its potential to address pressing unmet medical needs.

As computational methods continue to mature, their role in transforming early-phase drug discovery becomes increasingly evident. The Dyna-HeteroAttnDR framework presented in this chapter represents a step forward in this evolution, providing not only predictive accuracy but also biological insight, scalability, and translational relevance. This model lays the groundwork for future efforts aimed at fusing clinical, molecular, and systems-level data into unified pipelines for accelerated and targeted drug repurposing.

5.2 Methodology

5.2.1 Problem Definition

The drug-disease association prediction (DDAP) task involves estimating the potential therapeutic relevance between a given drug and a specific disease. Rather than being framed as a binary classification problem (i.e., associated or not), this task is modeled as a score regression problem, where the strength of the association is quantified on a continuous scale.

Let:

- $\mathcal{D} = \{\boldsymbol{d}_1, \boldsymbol{d}_2, \ldots, \boldsymbol{d}_\mathrm{m}\}$ represent the set of drugs, and
- $\mathcal{DS} = \{\boldsymbol{\delta}_1, \boldsymbol{\delta}_2, \ldots, \boldsymbol{\delta}_n\}$ denote the set of diseases.

The objective is to learn a mapping function:

$$g: (d_i, \delta_j) \to r_{ij}, r_{ij} \in [0,1]$$

where r_{ij} indicates the predicted association strength between drug d_i and disease δ_j. The interpretation of the score r_{ij} is as follows:

$$r_{ij} = \begin{cases} \text{Low Association,} & \text{if } r_{ij} < 0.5 \\ \text{Moderate Association,} & \text{if } 0.5 \leq r_{ij} \leq 0.8 \\ \text{High Association,} & \text{if } r_{ij} > 0.8 \end{cases}$$

5.2.2 Model Architecture

This section outlines the methodology used to predict drug–disease associations, emphasizing the framework's architecture and training procedure. The proposed model learns informative node representations from graph-based inputs by integrating both sparse and dense graph processing strategies. A key contribution of this approach is the incorporation of a hierarchical attention framework alongside fixed weight assignment, allowing the system to effectively learn and distinguish complex relational patterns within the network.

The hierarchical attention mechanism plays a crucial role by enabling the model to prioritize informative features within the graph across multiple layers. This layered attention approach incrementally builds node representations, refining them progressively from local to global perspectives. Each layer captures different levels of topological and semantic information, contributing to a more nuanced and comprehensive embedding. Static weight assignment complements this process by enabling a non-uniform weighting scheme across layers. This means that not all layers contribute equally; each layer's influence is modulated to optimize the learning of both localized and long-range structural information within the graph.

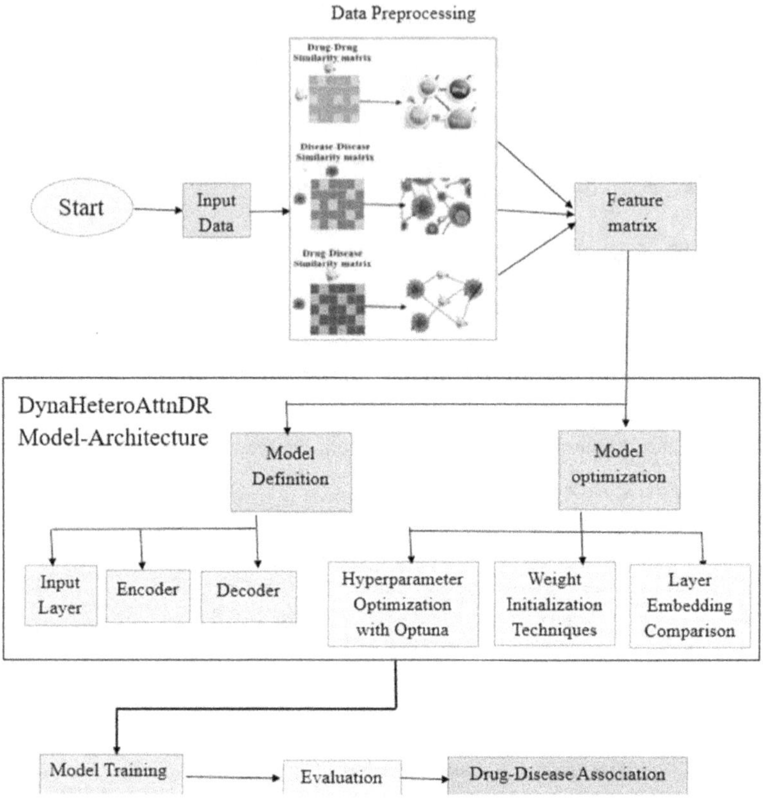

Figure 5.1: Proposed Methodology Framework

To achieve this, a Hybrid Deep Graph Attention Network is employed. This architecture is adept at encoding the diverse structural and semantic relationships inherent in drug-disease interaction networks. The model is designed to work with heterogeneous graphs, where different types of nodes (e.g., drugs and diseases) and different types of edges (e.g., interactions, similarities) are present. Figure 5.1 depicts the structure of the proposed approach. It is capable of learning from such mixed-type data by treating node types and edge types differently during the embedding process. The architecture comprises the following key components (i) Input Layer (ii) Encoder Module (iii) Decoder Module and (iv) Optimization Module. The proposed methodology integrates attention-based learning with heterogeneous graph structures to enable accurate and interpretable drug-disease association predictions. By leveraging both the structural diversity and semantic richness of biomedical networks, the model stands as a robust framework for advancing computational drug repurposing and disease targeting research.

5.2.2.1 Input layer

The input layer is essential for transforming raw biomedical data into a structure suitable for processing by a graph neural network. This layer receives a drug-disease adjacency matrix along with individual feature matrices for drugs and diseases, which collectively represent known associations and intrinsic attributes of the entities. Specifically, the focus lies in encoding the relationships between drugs and diseases using both association and similarity matrices. This process starts by integrating three primary input components, the drug-disease association matrix, which is a binary matrix of dimensions $N_{\text{drugs}} \times N_{\text{diseases}}$. An element $\mathcal{A}_{ij} = 1$ indicates a known therapeutic association between drug i and disease j, whereas $\mathcal{A}_{ij} = 0$ reflects no established link. Complementing this are two critical similarity matrices that capture intrinsic characteristics of drugs and diseases, ensuring the model integrates both relational knowledge and entity-specific features as the foundational input for subsequent representation learning.

- The drug similarity matrix Sd encodes pairwise similarities among drugs in a square format of size $N_{\text{drugs}} \times N_{\text{drugs}}$
- The disease similarity matrix St, a square matrix of size $N_{\text{diseases}} \times N_{\text{diseases}}$, quantifying how similar two diseases are based on biological or phenotypic features.

These matrices collectively serve as the foundation for constructing a heterogeneous graph that captures both intra- and inter-entity relationships. The adjacency matrix H of the heterogeneous graph is formulated as a feature matrix combining similarity and interaction data [137]. This matrix structure enables the unified representation of drugs and diseases as nodes in a graph, where edges signify either direct associations or similarity-based links, from Sd and St.

$$H = \begin{bmatrix} S_d & A \\ A^T & S_t \end{bmatrix}$$

Constructing the Heterogeneous Adjacency Matrix

To make this construction more concrete, consider a simple case with 3 drugs (D1, D2, D3) and 2 diseases (C1, C2).

1. Drug Similarity Matrix (3×3) :

$$\begin{bmatrix} 1.0 & 0.8 & 0.5 \\ 0.8 & 1.0 & 0.6 \\ 0.5 & 0.6 & 1.0 \end{bmatrix}$$

2. Disease Similarity Matrix (2×2):

$$\begin{bmatrix} 1.0 & 0.7 \\ 0.7 & 1.0 \end{bmatrix}$$

3. Drug-Disease Association Matrix (3×2):

$$\begin{bmatrix} 1 & 0 \\ 0 & 1 \\ 1 & 1 \end{bmatrix}$$

Using these, the combined adjacency matrix A of size 5×5 was constructed:

$$\begin{bmatrix} 1.0 & 0.8 & 0.5 & 1 & 0 \\ 0.8 & 1.0 & 0.6 & 0 & 1 \\ 0.5 & 0.6 & 1.0 & 1 & 1 \\ 1 & 0 & 1 & 1.0 & 0.7 \\ 0 & 1 & 1 & 0.7 & 1.0 \end{bmatrix}$$

Here:

- The top-left block is the drug-drug similarity matrix.
- The top-right block captures drug-disease interactions.
- The bottom-left is the transpose of the interaction matrix.
- The bottom-right block is the disease-disease similarity matrix.

This configuration builds a complete graph structure where each node (drug or disease) is connected based on either biological similarity or known interaction.

Generating the Feature Matrix

Unlike traditional GNN applications where node features might include molecular fingerprints (for drugs) or genetic markers (for diseases), the approach simplifies the process by using the graph structure itself as the basis for node features. The feature matrix X is directly derived from the adjacency matrix:

$$X = \begin{bmatrix} A & 0 \\ 0 & A^T \end{bmatrix}$$

Each row in X denotes a graph node, with values notates that node's relationship with others, thus encoding structural, association-based, and similarity-driven information. For example, the feature vector for drug D1 would look like:

$$[1.0,0.8,0.5,1,0]$$

indicating D1's self-similarity, similarity with D2 and D3, and associations with diseases C1 and C2.

Graph Normalization for Stability and Efficiency

To ensure effective learning during model training, normalization of the adjacency matrix is critical. This is done using the symmetric normalization rule, and the feature matrix generation is illustrated in Figure 5.2.

$$\tilde{A} = D^{-0.5}AD^{-0.5} \qquad (5.1)$$

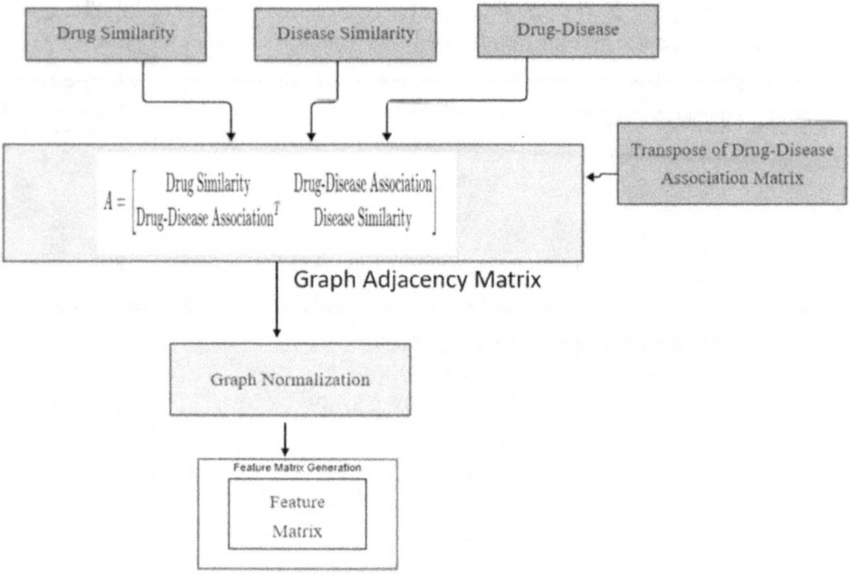

Figure 5.2: Feature Matrix Generation

Here, D is defined as the degree matrix, with diagonal entries equal to the sum of edge weights linked to each node. This operation scales the contributions of nodes based on their degree, helping to stabilize the learning process in GNNs and prevent exploding or vanishing gradients during training

5.2.2.2 Encoder

The encoder of the proposed framework employs a multi-layer heterogeneous graph attention mechanism to derive meaningful embeddings for nodes within the drug-disease heterogeneous bipartite graph (Figure 5.3). This design draws inspiration from prior work on Graph Convolutional Networks (GCNs) [138] and Graph Attention Networks (GATs) [139], but extends them to account for the heterogeneity inherent in biomedical networks, where drugs and diseases represent distinct node types connected by therapeutic associations and enriched with similarity information. Within each layer of the encoder, node representations are refined by selectively attending to their neighbors.

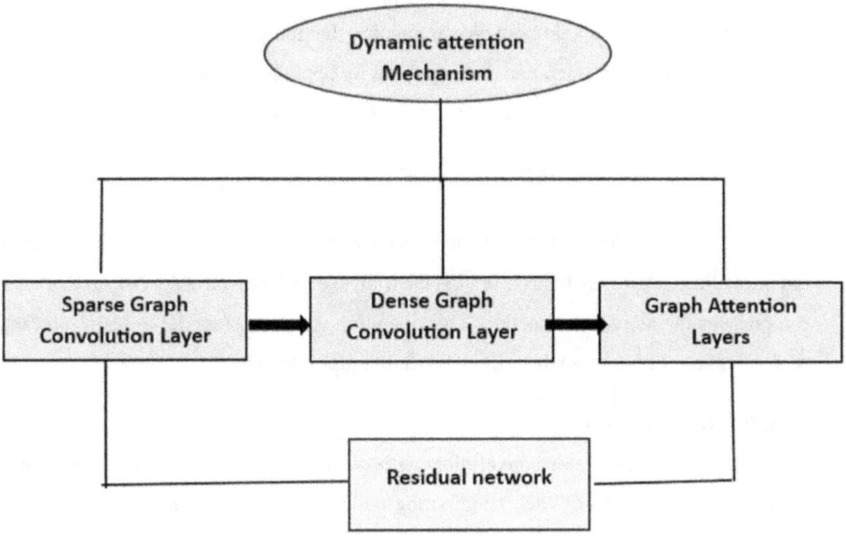

Figure 5.3: Encoder Architecture

The attention weights, or importance scores, are learned during training and enable the model to emphasize the most relevant interactions while diminishing noisy or less informative connections. In addition, a hierarchical attention mechanism is incorporated to ensure that both local and global structural contexts are preserved: immediate neighbors contribute localized relational knowledge, while higher-order dependencies across the network are progressively captured as the information propagates through multiple layers. By iteratively applying this process, the encoder produces embeddings that not only capture intrinsic features of nodes but also encode their contextual roles within the broader biomedical graph. The final output of this multi-layer heterogeneous attention encoder is therefore a set of task-optimized, context-aware embeddings that serve as robust inputs for the downstream prediction module.

Sparse Graph Convolution Layer

The sparse graph convolution layer is specifically designed to enable efficient computation on graphs with limited connectivity by operating directly on sparse adjacency matrices. As these graphs have substantially fewer edges than the maximum possible, the layer reduces computational complexity by processing only the non-zero elements of the adjacency matrix. This efficiency makes it well-suited for large-scale, real-world graph data.

To enhance generalization and avoid overfitting, dropout regularization is applied to the sparse adjacency matrix A, via a dropout sparse function that randomly omits edges during training. The graph convolution operation is carried out by applying a trainable weight matrix to the node features [140], enabling their transformation during learning.

$$H^{(l+1)} = \sigma\left(\tilde{A}H^{(l)}W^{(l)}\right) \qquad (5.2)$$

In this formulation, $H^{(l)}$ denotes the node feature representations at layer l, $\tilde{A}$ corresponds to the normalized adjacency matrix, $W^{(l)}$ is the trainable weight matrix specific to that layer, and σ represents the activation function. This operation enables the model to learn relevant node representations efficiently while accommodating graph sparsity.

Graph Attention Layers

This layer combines graph convolution with an attention-based approach that adaptively adjusts the significance of each neighboring node during feature aggregation [137]. Unlike GCNs, which apply equal weighting to connected nodes, GAT layers learn attention scores that reflect the relative importance of each connection. This permits the model to focus on more informative relationships, capturing intricate inter-node dependencies.

The final node representation results from a weighted sum across various attention heads and layers. The attention computation [141] is described by:

$$h'_i = \sigma\left(\sum_{j\in\mathcal{N}_i} \frac{\exp\left(a^T\cdot\max\left(Wh_i\|Wh_j,\alpha(Wh_i\|Wh_j)\right)\right)}{\sum_{k\in\mathcal{N}_i}\exp\left(a^T\cdot\max\left(Wh_i\|Wh_k,\alpha(Wh_i\|Wh_k)\right)\right)} Wh_j\right) \qquad (5.3)$$

Here, h'_i represents the updated node feature for node i, with h_i, h_j being the input features of node i and its neighbor j. W is a learnable transformation matrix, and a is a trainable attention vector determining the contribution of neighbors. This mechanism introduces both static and dynamic representation components, where GAT handles localized relevance and GCN addresses broader network connectivity.

Layer Normalization and Residual Networks

To further enhance performance and training stability, the design integrates layer normalization and residual connections into the architecture [142]. Layer normalization ensures consistent feature distributions across layers by normalizing activations, which stabilizes training dynamics and accelerates convergence. This is particularly beneficial in deep models, where shifts in activation scales can hinder learning progression.

Simultaneously, residual connections mitigate the issues of vanishing gradients, and over-smoothing is mitigated by reintroducing the layer's initial input to bypass transformations and be directly added to the output. This helps retain essential features throughout the network's depth. The formulation for residual learning is given by:

$$X^{(l+1)} = \mathrm{LayerNorm}\left(F\left(X^{(l)}\right)\right) + X^{(l)} \qquad (5.4)$$

Where $X^{(l)}$ is the input feature at layer l, and $F\left(X^{(l)}\right)$ represents the transformed feature after passing through the layer. LayerNorm denotes the normalization function applied prior to addition. This setup ensures improved gradient flow, facilitates the construction of deeper networks, and enhances the model's ability to generalize thereby increasing predictive accuracy for tasks such as identifying relevant drug-disease associations.

5.2.2.3 Decoder

Within the framework, the decoder serves as a critical bridge connecting the learned latent representations to the prediction of drug-disease interactions, specifically by generating the full drug-disease relationship matrix. An Inner Product Decoder [143], an efficient and computationally lightweight approach, was employed to model intrinsic relationships embedded in the representations. To improve the model's capacity to generalize and minimize overfitting tendencies, dropout regularization is applied during decoding. Subsequently, the learned embeddings are refined using a trainable weight matrix initialized via the Glorot scheme [144], which enhances their expressiveness before interaction estimation. Drug embeddings are then multiplied by the transposed disease embeddings, and a sigmoid activation function is applied to the resulting scores. This activation constrains the outputs within a probability range, making them suitable for interpretation as interaction likelihoods. The inner product operation, though parameter-efficient, offers a fast and effective means of computing similarity between entities. The resulting reconstructed scores are ultimately used to predict new drug-disease associations, playing a vital role in the broader objective of drug repurposing. The decoding approach recovers known links and reveals new therapeutic possibilities, aiding medical innovation.

5.2.3 Training and Optimization

To ensure optimal performance, the model is trained using a multi-faceted strategy that emphasizes efficiency, robustness, and generalization. The various optimization techniques employed are depicted in Figure 5.4. Additionally, the model is trained using the dataset described in Chapter 3 (Section 3.2).

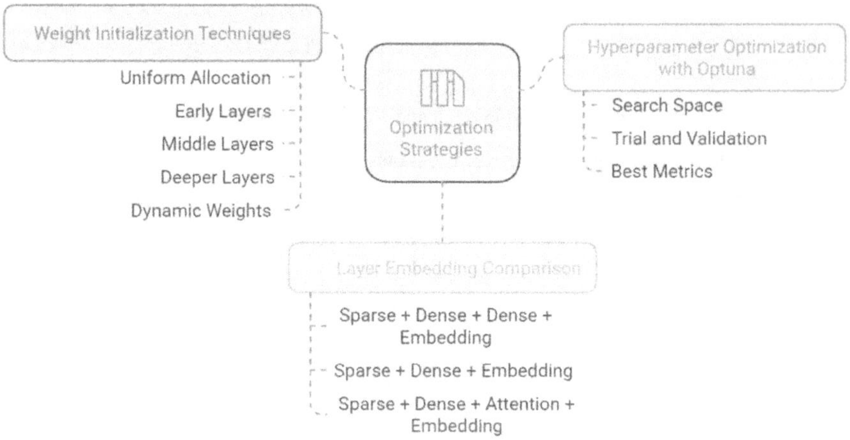

Figure 5.4: Optimization strategies

We utilize Optuna [145], a hyperparameter optimization tool, to systematically tune parameters such as learning rate, embedding size, dropout probability, and adjacency dropout rate [137]. This automated approach helps identify configurations that yield the best model performance. To prevent overfitting and validate the model's consistency, five-fold cross-validation is implemented across different dataset partitions. The model employs a modified cross-entropy loss that applies separate weights to positive and negative examples, improving training consistency. In addition, dropout is introduced at both the feature and graph structure levels to promote generalization and prevent overfitting [146]. Together, these complementary techniques result in a well-calibrated and resilient model that excels at capturing complex patterns within graph-based drug repurposing tasks.

5.2.3.1 Hyperparameter Optimization Strategy

To enhance model performance, this study employed Optuna, an advanced and efficient hyperparameter tuning library. The objective was to enhance the chosen metric by identifying the most effective set of hyperparameters. The parameters selected for optimization include the following:

- Embedding Size (emb_dim): Defines the size of the latent vector representations learned for both drug and disease nodes. The candidate values considered were 32, 64, 96, and 128, which represent progressively increasing levels of feature granularity, ranging from compact to higher-capacity embeddings.
- Learning Rate (lr): Specifies the step size for updating parameters during gradient descent. The search space was defined on a logarithmic scale from 1×10^{-4} to 1×10^{-2}, ensuring coverage of both small and relatively larger update steps.
- Dropout Rate (dp): Introduces regularization by randomly deactivating neurons during training to mitigate overfitting. The tested values were 0.2, 0.3, 0.4, 0.5, and 0.6, selected based on widely adopted ranges in deep learning literature and preliminary experiments showing stability within this interval.
- Adjacency Dropout Rate (adjdp): Applies dropout to the adjacency matrix to prevent over smoothing and encourage robustness in graph-based learning. The same range of values (0.2 to 0.6) was tested here, consistent with practices in graph neural network optimization.
- Number of Epochs: Denotes the number of complete training iterations. Candidate values of 200, 300, 400, 500, and 600 were explored, reflecting a balance between undertraining and computational efficiency.

A total of 50 optimization runs were performed, with each run subjected to 5-fold cross-validation to ensure result reliability. Among these, Trial 26 emerged as the best-performing configuration, achieving a top evaluation score of 0.3428. The fine-tuned hyperparameter settings are presented in Table 5.1.

Table 5.1: Optimal set of hyperparameters determined using Optuna

Hyperparameter	Optimal Value
Embedding Dimension (emb_dim)	96
Learning Rate (lr)	0.00745
Dropout Rate (dp)	0.3
Adjacency Dropout Rate (adjdp)	0.5
Epochs	500

5.2.3.2 Evaluation of Weight Initialization Techniques

Weight initialization is a critical factor influencing model convergence and overall performance. In this work, several strategies for initializing attention weights were tested, including Uniform Distribution, Emphasis on Initial Layers, Focus on Middle Layers, Deep Layer Prioritization, and Dynamic Attention Mechanism[147]. Each method was assessed using standard metrics such as AUPR, AUC, Accuracy, Recall, and Specificity. The experimental outcomes are summarized in Table 5.2.

1. Uniform Distribution (0.33, 0.33, 0.33): In this strategy, all layers are treated with the same attention weight. The results were consistent across metrics, but none achieved standout performance.

2. Early Layer Emphasis (0.6, 0.3, 0.1): Based on the assumption that early layers capture foundational features, this strategy aimed to improve generalizability. However, it did not yield significant gains, with both recall and precision showing minor reductions.

3. Middle Layer Priority (0.3, 0.5, 0.2): By prioritizing intermediate-layer representations, the method aimed to capture more informative feature interactions. However, despite modest improvements in AUC and recall, it resulted in lower precision and F1-score, reflecting a compromise in model performance

4. Deep Layer Emphasis (0.2, 0.3, 0.5): This technique focuses on deeper representations to boost abstract feature learning. Although precision and accuracy increased, the reduced recall implies that certain positive samples were not identified.

Table 5.2: Comparative Study of Weight Initialization Approaches

Initialization Strategy	AUPR	AUC	Accuracy	Recall	Specificity
Uniform Distribution (⅓, ⅓, ⅓).	0.3820	0.7314	0.5805	0.6925	0.5796
Initial Layer Priority (0.6, 0.3, 0.1)	0.3821	0.7310	0.5803	0.6904	0.5795
Prioritizing Middle Layers (0.3, 0.5, 0.2)	0.3816	0.7313	0.5799	0.6914	0.5790
Deeper Layer Priority (0.2, 0.3, 0.5)	0.3795	0.7319	0.5814	0.6815	0.5806
Dynamic Attention Weights	0.2830	0.8926	0.9729	0.4251	0.9773

5. Dynamic Attention Weights: Unlike fixed strategies, this approach learns the relative importance of each layer during training. It consistently outperformed all static methods, with an AUC of 0.8926, an Accuracy of 0.9729, and a Specificity of 0.9773. The findings suggest that the model effectively recognized which layers contribute most to learning meaningful representations.

To gain deeper insight into how different initialization methods influence the training process, the validation loss was monitored over multiple training epochs. The convergence patterns are visualized in Figure 5.5.

- Uniform and fixed strategies converged more slowly and required more epochs to stabilize.

- Dynamic Attention Weights led to faster convergence, achieving a stable validation loss in fewer epochs.

- This adaptability helped the model avoid suboptimal local minima, ultimately enhancing both speed and prediction quality.

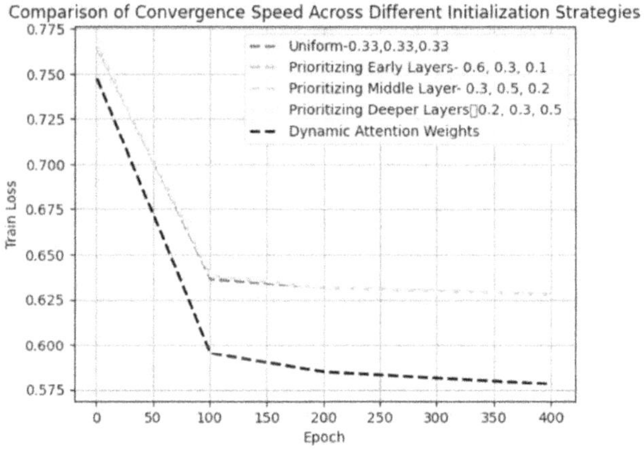

Figure 5.5: Convergence curve across different initialization strategies

Based on the experimental evidence, the Dynamic Attention Weighting mechanism is strongly recommended because of its:

- Superior performance across key metrics like AUC, accuracy, and specificity,

- Quicker convergence, reducing computational training time,

- Adaptive feature extraction, allowing efficient use of information from various depth layers.

The results suggest that allowing the model to learn the attention distribution dynamically, rather than depending on pre-assigned weightings, greatly boosts both predictive accuracy and model robustness.

5.2.3.3 Embedding Layer Configurations and Analysis

To systematically investigate the effect of different architectural designs on representation learning, three distinct configurations were developed. Each configuration combines sparse convolutional layers, dense convolutional layers, and in one case an attention mechanism, with the goal of capturing drug-disease interaction patterns at multiple levels of granularity. The sparse convolutional layer was employed to efficiently process large, sparsely connected graphs by focusing only on non-zero entries of the adjacency matrix, thereby reducing computational overhead. Dense convolutional layers were then introduced to enable richer feature aggregation across all available connections, enhancing the model's capacity to learn complex structural dependencies. Finally, an attention mechanism was incorporated in one configuration to dynamically assign higher importance to the most informative neighbors, further enhancing the expressiveness of the learned embeddings. The purpose of these configurations was to evaluate how variations in depth and mechanism (sparse vs. dense vs. attention) influence embedding quality and reconstruction accuracy. Detailed descriptions of each configuration, including their specific layer arrangements and embedding strategies, are provided in the following sections.

Configuration A: Sparse → Dense → Dense → Embedding

This setup initiates with a graph convolution layer optimized for sparse connectivity, followed by two densely connected graph convolution layers. An embedding layer concludes the sequence. A normalization step is applied after the second dense layer to stabilize the learning process. The resulting node representations are obtained by computing a weighted aggregate of outputs from each intermediate layer. Reconstruction is handled through an Inner Product Decoder.

Configuration B: Sparse → Dense → Embedding

This variation simplifies the previous design by removing one dense layer, resulting in a more compact and efficient architecture. As in the first setup, the final embedding is generated by combining the intermediate representations through a weighted summation.

Table 5.3: Comparative evaluation of performance metrics across all three architectural variants.

Sl no	Configuration	AUPR	AUC	Accuracy	Recall	Specificity
1	Sparse Convolution + Conv + Conv + Emb	0.2694	0.8772	0.9723	0.4106	0.9768
2	Sparse Convolution + Conv + Emb	0.2701	0.878	0.9724	0.4074	0.977
3	Sparse Convolution + Conv + Attention + Emb	0.283	0.8945	0.9856	0.4251	0.9913

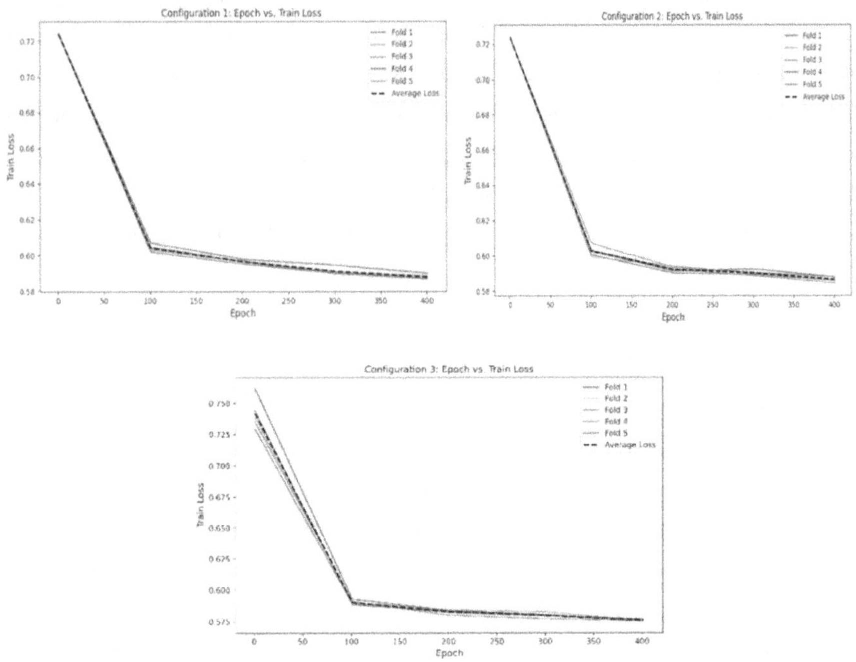

Figure 5.6 (a-c): Training loss over epochs for five cross-validation folds. (a) Configuration 1, (b) Configuration 2, and (c) Configuration 3.

Configuration C: Sparse → Dense → Attention → Embedding

This design integrates an attention module immediately after the dense convolutional layer. The attention mechanism enables adaptive weighting, allowing the model to emphasize important features within the graph structure. The final representation is computed by fusing the outputs of the sparse, dense, and attention layers, thereby enriching the quality of the learned embedding.

The performance outcomes for all three configurations are summarized in Table 5.3. Among them, Configuration C demonstrated superior results across all evaluation metrics due to the integration of the attention mechanism. Specifically, the AUPR and AUC scores increased by 5.06% and 1.83%, respectively, when compared with Configuration A.

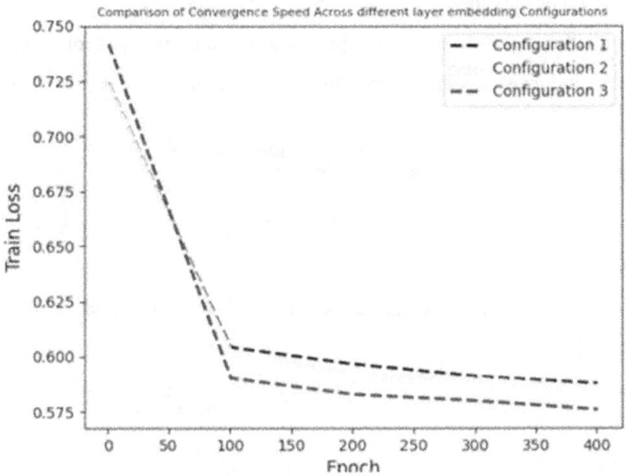

Figure 5.6: Convergence trends across various embedding layer settings

Configurations A and B performed comparably, indicating that the additional dense convolutional layer in Configuration A did not provide significant improvements over the leaner Configuration B. The results suggest that the incorporation of attention in Configuration C significantly enhanced performance by effectively extracting salient features from the graph structure. This justifies integrating attention-based strategies into GNNs to address the precision and accuracy requirements of certain tasks. Figures 5.6 illustrate the training loss over epochs curve for five cross-validation folds, as well as the average loss. In figure 5.6, the solid lines represent individual folds, while the dashed line indicates the average loss across folds. To further evaluate how different embedding strategies influence training efficiency, their convergence behavior was analyzed. This is visualized in Figure 5.7, where validation loss curves are plotted over epochs.

5.3 Evaluation Metrics

Various evaluation metrics are applied to examine the model's effectiveness across multiple dimensions. These include:

AUC (Area under the ROC Curve)

This metric quantifies the region beneath the ROC curve, which contrasts the proportion of correctly identified positives with the proportion of incorrectly identified positives. A greater AUC value indicates stronger capability in distinguishing between negative and positive classes

$$TPR = \frac{TP}{TP+FN} \tag{5.4}$$

$$FPR = \frac{FP}{FP+TN} \tag{5.5}$$

F1 Score

The F1 score represents the harmonic mean of precision and recall, and is expressed mathematically as:

$$F1 = 2 * \frac{Precision * Recall}{Precision + Recall} \tag{5.6}$$

Accuracy

Accuracy represents the proportion of accurately identified cases (including both positives and negatives) out of the overall number of predictions made:

$$Accuracy = \frac{TP+TN}{TP+TN+FP+FN} \tag{5.7}$$

Specificity

Specificity reflects the model's capacity to correctly identify negative associations, i.e., distinguishing non-interacting drug-disease pairs

$$Specificity = \frac{TN}{TN+FP} \tag{5.8}$$

Recall

Also referred to as sensitivity, recall quantifies the proportion of actual positive instances that are successfully detected by the model.

$$Recall = \frac{TP}{TP+} \tag{5.9}$$

A higher recall score suggests the model is proficient at capturing relevant drug-disease associations, minimizing the chance of missing true positives.

5.4 Results and Analysis

To rigorously assess the stability of the model, a five-part cross-validation strategy was adopted. In each iteration, the matrix representing drug-disease associations was divided into separate training and evaluation segments. Approximately 80% of the entries were randomly assigned to the training set, while the remaining 20% were allocated for validation. A consistent random seed was used to shuffle indices, ensuring reproducibility and minimizing sampling bias. For each partition, evaluation metrics were computed and then averaged across all folds to obtain a reliable measure of the model's effectiveness. Figure 5.8 explains the evaluation metric scores of the proposed model.

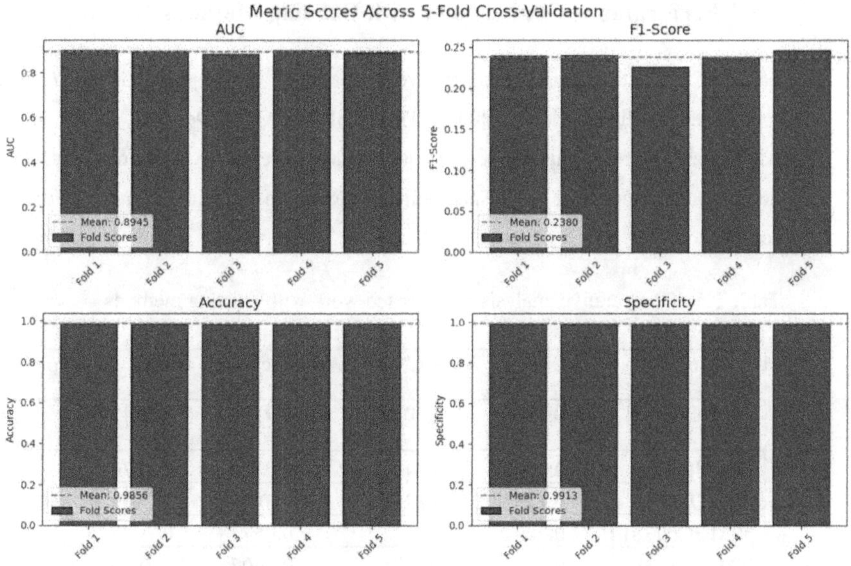

Figure 5.7: Evaluation metrics scores of the proposed model

The proposed framework incorporates optimized hyperparameters identified through Optuna and combines both sparse and dense graph convolution techniques with an adaptive attention mechanism. This integration enhances the model's ability to extract and prioritize meaningful features. Final node representations are derived by aggregating the outputs from the convolution and attention components using a learnable weighting strategy. Table 5.4 presents the cross-validation results, where the model achieved an AUC of 0.8945, demonstrating its effectiveness in class discrimination. Its accuracy of 98.56% and specificity of 99.13% further indicate excellent performance in correctly identifying negative instances. However, the harmonic mean of precision and recall, calculated at 0.238, reflects the inherent trade-offs involved in balancing various performance indicators.

Table 5.4: Evaluation results for the proposed framework

Metric	AUPR	AUC	F1 Score	Accuracy	Recall	Specificity
Value	0.283	0.8945	0.238	0.9856	0.4251	0.9913

5.4.1 Performance Comparison with Existing Methods

Table 5.5 presents a detailed comparative evaluation of the proposed method against a set of established baseline models, including TL-HGBI, NIMGCN, DeepDR, DRRS, and LAGCN. All models were rigorously assessed using widely accepted evaluation metrics such as F1-Score, AUPR, Accuracy, AUC, Specificity, and Recall to ensure a comprehensive performance comparison.

Table 5.5: Comparative analysis of proposed work with existing methods

Model	AUPR	AUC	Accuracy	Recall	Specificity
TL-HGBI[35]	0.0665	0.7029	0.9114	0.2545	0.9284
DRRS[36]	0.1321	0.8429	0.9324	0.3276	0.9468
DeepDR[37]	0.1351	0.8211	0.94	0.2959	0.9567
NIMGCN[38]	0.2002	0.8533	0.9572	0.3083	0.9739
LAGCN[33]	0.3168	0.875	0.9605	0.36	0.976
Our Model	0.283	**0.8945**	**0.9856**	**0.4251**	**0.9913**

The proposed approach attained the highest accuracy of 98.56% and specificity of 99.13%, surpassing all other models in these metrics. Notably, LAGCN yielded the best AUPR, registering a value of 0.3168. These results emphasize the strength and reliability of the proposed framework, demonstrating its superior performance over existing methods and its effectiveness for the targeted prediction task.

5.4.2 Experiment Validation

One of the major challenges in modern medicine is the effective treatment of rare diseases, which collectively affect millions of people worldwide [148]. The European Union classifies a disease as rare when it affects fewer than one person in every two thousand. Despite their collective impact, these conditions remain significantly underserved due to limited research funding, scarce therapeutic development, and often delayed diagnoses [149]. More than 7,000 rare diseases have been identified to date, yet the majority lack approved treatments, leaving patients with few or no viable options.

This situation is further compounded by the high cost and extended durations required for traditional drug discovery, making it commercially unviable for pharmaceutical companies to invest heavily in treatments for small patient populations. Consequently, many patients with rare diseases face a grim reality where life-saving therapies remain out of reach, not only due to scientific limitations but also economic and systemic hurdles.

Within this framework, repositioning existing pharmaceuticals stands out as both an efficient and impactful approach. It involves uncovering alternative therapeutic applications for approved compounds by building on existing knowledge of their safety profiles, absorption characteristics, and pharmacological actions [150]. This strategy substantially lowers the development cost, timeline, and associated risks compared to de novo drug discovery. Importantly, repurposed drugs often bypass early-phase clinical trials, accelerating their path to patient access. For rare diseases, where time is critical and therapeutic gaps are immense, drug repurposing offers a feasible route to address unmet clinical needs.

Recognizing this potential, the present study extends its trained predictive model, originally developed to learn complex drug-disease interactions, towards the task of drug repurposing for rare diseases. This model, with its capability to capture intricate biological associations through multi-layer representation learning and attention mechanisms, is particularly well-suited for rare diseases. These conditions are often characterized by heterogeneous phenotypes, immune system involvement, and multi-organ effects, which align with the model's strengths in handling multidimensional biomedical data[151]. Accordingly, a unified experimental framework was established, wherein the model was systematically evaluated across four representative rare diseases to ensure consistency and comparability of predictions.

- Churg-Strauss Syndrome (Eosinophilic Granulomatosis with Polyangiitis, EGPA)
- Cystic Fibrosis
- Glioblastoma
- Burkitt Lymphoma

These diseases were selected based on shared features such as inflammatory or oncogenic profiles, limited therapeutic options, and existing gaps in current treatment paradigms, which make them ideal candidates for a repurposing-driven approach. For each condition, the model generated a ranked list of drugs predicted to be associated with therapeutic potential, grounded in learned biological relevance rather than random associations.

The subsequent subsections delve into each disease, presenting the predicted repurposed drugs, current treatment limitations, and how the identified candidates align with or extend existing therapeutic insights. This step marks a crucial phase in bridging computational predictions with clinical utility, demonstrating how intelligent models can assist in discovering novel uses for known compounds in underrepresented disease spaces.

5.4.2.1 Churg-Strauss Syndrome (EGPA, Eosinophilic Granulomatosis with Polyangiitis)

Churg-Strauss Syndrome, also referred to as Eosinophilic Granulomatosis with Polyangiitis (EGPA), is a rare but clinically significant autoimmune vasculitis that affects multiple organ systems. It is characterized by inflammation of small to medium-sized blood vessels and is distinguished by a marked increase in eosinophils, a subset of immune cells central to allergic and inflammatory responses. This pathological immune dysregulation results in widespread tissue injury, often manifesting in the lungs, skin, heart, gastrointestinal tract, and peripheral nervous system. Patients typically present with a highly variable clinical spectrum that may include severe asthma, chronic sinusitis, allergic rhinitis, peripheral neuropathy, cutaneous lesions, and cardiac dysfunction. This heterogeneity complicates both early diagnosis and long-term disease management.

From an epidemiological perspective, EGPA is extremely rare, with an estimated incidence of only 1-4 cases per million annually, yet the disease carries significant morbidity due to organ-threatening complications. Current diagnostic frameworks, such as the American College of Rheumatology (ACR) criteria, emphasize the coexistence of asthma, eosinophilia, neuropathy, pulmonary infiltrates, and biopsy-proven vasculitis. However, because of its overlap with other systemic autoimmune diseases, EGPA remains diagnostically challenging, often leading to delays in initiating appropriate therapy.

Table 5.6: Predicted Drugs for Churg-Strauss Syndrome (EGPA)

Drug	Score	Evidence	Other Main Diseases Treated
Prednisolone	0.9994	A corticosteroid that suppresses the immune system and reduces inflammation; the cornerstone of EGPA treatment due to control of blood vessel inflammation [152].	Asthma, Rheumatoid Arthritis, Systemic Lupus Erythematosus
Methotrexate	0.9992	Immunosuppressants are used for EGPA treatment, especially for patients intolerant to corticosteroids. It reduces relapses and allows corticosteroid dose reduction [153].	Rheumatoid Arthritis, Psoriasis, Burkitt Lymphoma
Phenytoin	0.9990	Anticonvulsant used in EGPA to manage peripheral neuropathy, a common complication; also possesses anti-inflammatory properties relevant to neurological symptoms [154].	Epilepsy, Neuropathic Pain
Carbamazepine	0.9979	Anticonvulsant with repurposing potential due to its neurological involvement in EGPA. It also has anti-inflammatory effects that may help manage EGPA-associated neurological symptoms [155].	Epilepsy, Bipolar Disorder
Methylprednisolone	0.9975	Corticosteroids are used to treat inflammation in EGPA. Effective in managing EGPA symptoms due to its potent anti-inflammatory action [152].	Asthma, Allergic Reactions, Rheumatoid Arthritis

Prednisone	0.9924	Widely used corticosteroid for EGPA treatment; reduces inflammation by suppressing the immune response [152].	Asthma, Inflammatory Bowel Disease
Valproic Acid	0.9888	Known for neurological conditions, it has anti-inflammatory properties that may be useful for managing neurological aspects of EGPA [156].	Epilepsy, Bipolar Disorder, Migraine
Cytarabine	0.9683	Chemotherapy drug with the potential to suppress abnormal immune responses in severe or resistant cases of EGPA [157].	Leukemia, Burkitt Lymphoma

Current treatment approaches predominantly rely on systemic corticosteroids, which remain the first-line therapy to control acute inflammation. In more severe or refractory cases, immunosuppressive agents such as cyclophosphamide, azathioprine, or methotrexate are employed. More recently, biological therapies targeting interleukin-5 (e.g., mepolizumab) have shown promise, given the central role of eosinophils in disease pathology. Nevertheless, treatment outcomes are inconsistent: some patients achieve long-term remission, while others experience frequent relapses or develop progressive organ damage despite therapy. Prolonged use of corticosteroids can cause considerable adverse outcomes, emphasizing the demand for alternative therapeutic options.

The rarity and complexity of EGPA make it a compelling candidate for drug repurposing research. By leveraging computational models capable of integrating gene expression, pathway involvement, and immunological interactions, new therapeutic opportunities can be uncovered more efficiently than through traditional drug discovery pipelines. In this study, the predictive neuro-symbolic framework was applied to EGPA to identify FDA-approved drugs with potential repurposing value.

The resulting predictions are summarized in Table 5.6, which provides a multi-dimensional view of candidate drugs. The 'Drug' column lists compounds prioritized by the model, while the 'Score' column reflects the predicted strength of association between the drug and EGPA. The 'Evidence' column links computational predictions to supporting biomedical literature, including mechanistic pathways or previously reported immunological relevance. Finally, the 'Other Main Diseases Treated' column highlights the existing indications of each candidate, thereby reinforcing the translational feasibility of repurposing them for EGPA.

Importantly, the framework not only rediscovered standard-of-care therapies, such as corticosteroids and immunosuppressants, validating the model's reliability, but also identified novel candidates with strong immunological or neurological relevance. Some predicted drugs have primary indications in allergic disorders, autoimmune diseases, or neurological syndromes, aligning closely with EGPA's multisystem nature. Others are approved for conditions where immune modulation and anti-inflammatory effects are central, further supporting their potential role in EGPA management.

By combining computational prediction, literature validation, and clinical feasibility assessment, the proposed framework highlights a set of promising therapeutic candidates that can guide future experimental studies and early-phase clinical trials. Given the scarcity of effective long-term treatments for EGPA, these predictions underscore the power of drug repurposing to bridge current therapeutic gaps, reduce reliance on broad immunosuppression, and ultimately improve patient outcomes.

5.4.2.2 Burkitt Lymphoma

Burkitt Lymphoma (BL) is a highly aggressive malignancy belonging to the group of B-cell non-Hodgkin lymphomas, recognized for its rapid proliferation rate and distinct biological features. It is among the fastest-growing human cancers, with untreated tumors capable of doubling in size within 24 to 48 hours. Clinically, BL is categorized into three major subtypes: endemic, primarily associated with Epstein-Barr virus (EBV) infection and most prevalent in equatorial Africa; sporadic, which occurs worldwide and frequently involves abdominal organs; and immunodeficiency-associated, often observed in individuals with HIV/AIDS or those undergoing immunosuppressive therapy. Despite their geographical and etiological distinctions, all forms share a common hallmark dysregulation of the MYC oncogene through chromosomal translocations, leading to uncontrolled cell cycle progression and heightened metabolic activity.

Owing to its biological aggressiveness, Burkitt Lymphoma demands immediate diagnosis and prompt therapeutic intervention. Current treatment strategies rely on intensive, multi-agent chemotherapy regimens, often incorporating methotrexate, cyclophosphamide, vincristine, cytarabine, doxorubicin, and rituximab. While such regimens have achieved high cure rates in pediatric and young adult populations, treatment outcomes in older patients remain suboptimal due to therapy-related toxicities. Moreover, relapsed or refractory cases continue to present significant clinical challenges, with survival rates dropping drastically once frontline therapy fails. The toxicity of high-dose chemotherapy, coupled with the emergence of resistance, underscores the urgent need for alternative and less toxic therapeutic approaches.

The inclusion of Burkitt Lymphoma in this study is thus both clinically and scientifically justified. Its unique molecular profile, driven predominantly by MYC dysregulation, rapid proliferation pathways, and reliance on DNA replication machinery, renders it particularly well suited for drug repurposing investigations. Repurposing existing FDA-approved drugs provides a pragmatic strategy for expanding the therapeutic arsenal, given the pressing clinical urgency associated with BL and the feasibility of translating already-approved compounds into clinical settings without lengthy preclinical development.

In the present study, a graph-based predictive model was applied to Burkitt Lymphoma datasets to identify repurposing opportunities. The model generated a ranked list of drug candidates based on predicted therapeutic relevance. Notably, established chemotherapeutics, including methotrexate, cytarabine, doxorubicin, and vincristine, were among the top-ranked predictions. The inclusion of these well-validated agents provides strong internal validation of the model's predictive robustness. In parallel, the model identified novel candidates such as paclitaxel, fluorouracil, and tretinoin, agents not routinely employed in BL but mechanistically aligned with its biology. For instance, paclitaxel's microtubule stabilization properties and fluorouracil's inhibition of nucleotide synthesis may disrupt the rapid mitotic activity characteristic of BL cells, while tretinoin's differentiation-inducing effects could counteract MYC-driven proliferation.

Table 5.7 presents these prioritized drugs along with their associated prediction scores, mechanistic or literature-based evidence, and existing clinical indications. The table serves as both a validation of the model by successfully recovering established standards of care and a platform for identifying unconventional candidates with potential translational value.

Table 5.7: Predicted Drugs for Burkitt Lymphoma

Drug	Score	Evidence	Other Main Diseases Treated
Methotrexate	1.0000	Methotrexate inhibits dihydrofolate reductase, blocking DNA synthesis in rapidly dividing cells. It is currently used in high doses for treating Burkitt Lymphoma as part of combination chemotherapy regimens [158].	Rheumatoid arthritis, Psoriasis, Osteosarcoma
Cytarabine	1.0000	Cytarabine falls under the category of pyrimidine nucleoside analogs, interfering with DNA synthesis and hence is suitable for the treatment of blood cancers, including Burkitt Lymphoma. Cytarabine has been used in combination with cyclophosphamide and rituximab for the treatment of Burkitt lymphoma, with high response rates [159].	Acute Myeloid Leukemia, Non-Hodgkin Lymphoma
Doxorubicin	1.0000	Doxorubicin is an anthracycline antibiotic that intercalates nucleic acids, thereby inhibiting macromolecular biosynthesis and topoisomerase II, an enzyme that provides for the proper segregation of DNA during replication and repair in cancer cells [160,161].	Breast Cancer, Ovarian Cancer, Hodgkin's Lymphoma
Vincristine	1.0000	Vincristine is a vinca alkaloid that disrupts microtubule formation, arresting cancer cell division. It is widely used in hematologic malignancies, including Burkitt Lymphoma [161].	Acute Lymphoblastic Leukemia, Hodgkin's Lymphoma

Paclitaxel	1.0000	Paclitaxel stabilizes microtubules and inhibits cell division. Although primarily used for solid tumors, it has shown potential in treating other aggressive malignancies, and could be considered for Burkitt Lymphoma [162].	Ovarian Cancer, Breast Cancer, Non-Small Cell Lung Cancer
Fluorouracil	0.9997	Fluorouracil is a pyrimidine analogue that inhibits thymidylate synthetase, which is an important enzyme in DNA replication. Although not a standard drug in the treatment of lymphoma, it is indeed an active candidate for further investigations in Burkitt Lymphoma, according to its mechanism of action [163].	Colorectal Cancer, Stomach Cancer, Breast Cancer
Prednisolone	0.9989	A corticosteroid is used to modulate the immune response and inflammation. It is commonly part of combination therapies in lymphomas and leukemias, including Burkitt Lymphoma [164].	Inflammatory Diseases, Allergic Disorders, Leukemia
Dexamethasone	0.9988	Dexamethasone is a potent corticosteroid with anti-inflammatory properties. It is frequently used in cancer therapy to reduce inflammation and edema, particularly in lymphoid cancers [161].	Multiple Myeloma, Brain Tumors, Inflammatory Conditions
Prednisone	0.9984	Prednisone, similar to prednisolone, is used in various lymphomas as part of multi-drug chemotherapy regimens. It suppresses the immune system and inflammation, aiding in the treatment of cancers such as Burkitt Lymphoma [163].	Autoimmune Diseases, Leukemia, Inflammatory Disorders

The findings suggest that repurposed agents may be rationally integrated into novel therapeutic combinations, potentially reducing chemotherapy intensity while maintaining efficacy.

Overall, the predictions underscore the dual capacity of the proposed framework: (i) to confirm established treatment paradigms, thereby demonstrating reliability, and (ii) to highlight repurposing leads that merit further experimental and clinical evaluation. By leveraging computational predictions anchored in biological plausibility, this approach offers a pathway to addressing the critical unmet needs in Burkitt Lymphoma, particularly for patients who relapse or cannot tolerate existing regimens. Ultimately, the integration of drug repurposing strategies may contribute to more effective, less toxic, and more personalized interventions for this high-risk lymphoma subtype.

5.4.2.3 Glioblastoma (GBM)

Glioblastoma (GBM) is the most common and malignant form of primary brain tumor in adults, representing approximately 45-50% of all gliomas. Classified as a World Health Organization (WHO) grade IV astrocytoma, GBM is characterized by rapid cellular proliferation, diffuse infiltration into surrounding brain tissue, and an extraordinary capacity to evade conventional therapies. Despite aggressive treatment combining surgical removal, radiotherapy, and temozolomide chemotherapy, the disease generally has a poor prognosis, with median survival usually limited to about 12–15 months. Long-term survival beyond five year remains dismally low, at less than 5%, underscoring the urgent and unmet need for innovative therapeutic strategies.

Several factors account for the dismal prognosis of GBM. First, its highly infiltrative nature means that microscopic tumor cells often extend beyond surgically accessible margins, making complete resection virtually impossible. Second, GBM exhibits profound intratumoral heterogeneity, with multiple subclones differing in genetic alterations, signaling pathways, and treatment sensitivities coexisting within a single tumor. This heterogeneity contributes significantly to treatment resistance and tumor recurrence. Third, the blood-brain barrier (BBB) represents a formidable obstacle, preventing adequate concentrations of many systemic drugs from reaching the tumor site. Furthermore, the tumor microenvironment, characterized by immunosuppressive cytokines, hypoxia, and aberrant vasculature, fosters an ecosystem that actively resists both immunotherapeutic and chemotherapeutic interventions.

Table 5.8: Predicted Drugs for Glioblastoma

Drug	Score	Evidence	Other Main Diseases Treated
Methotrexate	1.0000	Antimetabolite used in cancer therapy; has been explored for GBM treatment in combination with other drugs [165].	Rheumatoid arthritis, psoriasis, other cancers (leukemia, osteosarcoma)
Dexamethasone	1.0000	Glucocorticoids are used to reduce brain swelling in GBM patients[166].	Inflammatory conditions, cerebral edema, and multiple sclerosis
Doxorubicin	1.0000	Chemotherapeutic agent that has limited use in GBM due to poor blood-brain barrier penetration [167].	Breast cancer, leukemia, and lymphoma
Tretinoin	1.0000	Has been shown to inhibit GBM cell proliferation in preclinical studies [168].	Acute promyelocytic leukemia
Aspirin	0.9999	Anti-inflammatory agent; studies suggest potential use in GBM due to its anti-tumor properties [169].	Cardiovascular disease, prevention of stroke, colorectal cancer
Fluorouracil	0.9996	Antimetabolite used in various cancers, with limited data on GBM efficacy [170].	Colorectal cancer, breast cancer, and pancreatic cancer
Indomethacin	0.9993	NSAID with some preclinical evidence of effectiveness against GBM cell lines[171].	Pain, inflammation, rheumatoid arthritis
Phenobarbital	0.9983	Antiepileptic drug used in GBM patients to control seizures [172].	Epilepsy, anxiety disorders, sedative
Tamoxifen	0.9982	Hormonal therapy is primarily used in breast cancer, with preclinical studies suggesting potential GBM benefit [173,174]	Breast cancer, endometrial cancer

Given these challenges, the selection of GBM for experimental validation within this study is particularly justified. Traditional drug discovery approaches, which typically span over a decade from early development to clinical approval, are inadequate in the face of such urgent clinical need. Drug repurposing, by contrast, leverages the existing safety, pharmacokinetic, and pharmacodynamic profiles of approved drugs, thereby offering a faster and more cost-effective pathway to novel therapeutic options. The capacity to reposition existing agents also provides an opportunity to identify drugs capable of modulating specific vulnerabilities of GBM, including pathways involved in cell cycle regulation, apoptosis, angiogenesis, and epigenetic remodeling.

Application of the trained predictive model to GBM datasets identified a panel of high-priority repurposing candidates with translational potential. Among the top-ranked drugs were methotrexate, dexamethasone, doxorubicin, and tretinoin, all of which exhibit mechanisms that align with the biological hallmarks of GBM. Methotrexate, an antimetabolite, has the potential to disrupt nucleotide synthesis in rapidly dividing glioblastoma cells. Dexamethasone, although primarily used for symptomatic relief of cerebral edema, has demonstrated immunomodulatory and anti-proliferative effects in glioma contexts. Doxorubicin, a DNA intercalating agent, is of particular interest given its established anti-cancer activity, though challenges related to permeability remain to be addressed through innovative delivery systems. Tretinoin, a retinoic acid derivative, exerts differentiation-inducing and pro-apoptotic effects, which could counteract the stem-like cell subpopulations thought to drive GBM recurrence.

Additionally, the model highlighted compounds such as aspirin and tamoxifen, drugs with well-documented safety profiles in other indications. Aspirin has shown promise in preclinical models of GBM through its ability to inhibit cyclooxygenase-mediated inflammatory pathways and potentially modulate tumor microenvironmental factors. Tamoxifen, widely used in breast cancer, has been reported to exert anti-glioma effects via protein kinase C inhibition and apoptosis induction. These examples illustrate the ability of the predictive framework not only to recover existing therapeutic mainstays but also to nominate unconventional agents with plausible mechanistic relevance.

Table 5.8 provides a summary of these predicted drugs, including model-assigned confidence scores, literature-based evidence, and primary indications in other diseases. Collectively, these results demonstrate the utility of the proposed approach in identifying both validated and novel candidates for GBM therapy. While further experimental and clinical validation is essential, these findings reinforce the promise of computational repurposing as a means of addressing one of the most challenging cancers in neuro-oncology.

5.4.2.4 Cystic Fibrosis

Cystic Fibrosis (CF) is an inherited condition caused by mutations in the CFTR (Cystic Fibrosis Transmembrane Conductance Regulator) gene, mainly impacting the lungs and digestive system. These mutations impair chloride and water transport across epithelial cell membranes, leading to the production of thick, viscous mucus that obstructs airways and ducts. In the respiratory system, this accumulation predisposes patients to chronic bacterial infections, persistent inflammation, and progressive lung damage, ultimately causing respiratory failure. In the digestive tract, mucus obstruction can lead to pancreatic insufficiency, malabsorption, and malnutrition. Beyond these primary systems, CF can impact the liver, sinuses, and reproductive organs, reflecting the multi-organ nature of the disease. Despite significant advances in clinical management, including airway clearance techniques, antibiotic therapies, and CFTR modulators such as ivacaftor and lumacaftor, CF remains a life-limiting condition, with many patients experiencing reduced life expectancy and persistent morbidity.

The inclusion of CF for experimental validation in this study is particularly important for several reasons. Firstly, CF represents a model rare disease where chronic inflammation, immune dysregulation, and multi-organ involvement are central to pathology, making it ideal for evaluating computational repurposing approaches. Secondly, while CFTR modulators have revolutionized care for some patients, a significant proportion, especially those carrying rare or complex CFTR mutations, derive limited or no benefit. Thirdly, the long-term medical burden of CF, including frequent hospitalizations, chronic pharmacotherapy, and intensive supportive care, imposes substantial economic and quality-of-life challenges, emphasizing the urgent need for novel or supplementary therapeutic strategies. Drug repurposing offers a pragmatic solution, enabling the identification of existing pharmacological agents with potential efficacy in CF, thereby bypassing the high costs and extended timelines associated with new drug development.

Application of the trained predictive model to CF datasets generated a prioritized list of candidate drugs with high potential for repurposing. These candidates were selected based on their biological relevance to CF pathology, including mechanisms that may reduce inflammation, improve mucus clearance, or mitigate secondary complications such as bacterial colonization. Several of these agents have demonstrated anti-inflammatory or muco-regulatory properties in preclinical studies or related disease contexts, suggesting plausible mechanistic support for their utility in CF management.

Table 5.9: Predicted Drugs for Cystic Fibrosis

Drug	Score	Evidence	Other Main Diseases Treated
Prednisolone	0.9351	Corticosteroids are used for inflammation. Limited evidence for CF, but may help manage exacerbations [175].	Asthma, Rheumatoid Arthritis, Crohn's Disease
Aspirin	0.9277	NSAID with anti-inflammatory properties. Shown to reduce lung inflammation in preclinical CF models [176].	Cardiovascular Diseases, Pain Management
Indomethacin	0.7964	NSAIDs that may reduce inflammation in CF, though evidence is limited to animal models [177].	Gout, Osteoarthritis, Rheumatoid Arthritis
Methylprednisolone	0.7046	Corticosteroids are used short-term in CF for reducing inflammation during exacerbations [178].	Multiple Sclerosis, Severe Allergic Reactions
Enalapril	0.6399	ACE inhibitors are speculated to help manage cardiovascular issues in advanced CF [179].	Hypertension, Heart Failure
Prednisone	0.5965	Corticosteroids are used for short-term inflammation control in CF, with concerns about long-term use [178].	Asthma, Autoimmune Diseases

The predicted drugs encompass compounds approved for respiratory, gastrointestinal, and immunological disorders, reflecting the multi-systemic nature of CF. For instance, drugs with known anti-inflammatory activity may help reduce chronic pulmonary inflammation, whereas agents affecting ion transport or cellular hydration could improve airway and ductal function. Importantly, these candidates exhibit established safety and pharmacokinetic profiles, which enhance their translational feasibility and position them as immediate candidates for experimental validation.

Table 5.9 summarizes the predicted repurposable drugs, the supporting evidence for their potential use in CF, and their primary indications in other diseases. Collectively, these findings illustrate the capacity of computational repurposing frameworks to identify both validated and novel therapeutic opportunities, offering a pathway to supplement existing CF treatments, address unmet clinical needs, and potentially improve patient outcomes. By integrating molecular, pharmacological, and disease-specific data, the model provides a rational foundation for future experimental studies and early-phase clinical investigations, emphasizing the value of drug repurposing in rare, high-burden diseases such as cystic fibrosis.

5.5 Conclusion

This chapter introduced an innovative approach for predicting drug-disease associations by integrating both sparse and dense graph convolution layers with an adaptive attention mechanism. To enhance model performance, hyperparameters were fine-tuned using the Optuna optimization framework. A rigorous evaluation was conducted using a 5-fold cross-validation scheme to validate the model's effectiveness and generalizability. The experimental results affirm that the proposed method achieves outstanding performance, recording an AUC of 0.8945, an accuracy of 98.56%, and a specificity of 99.13%.

The integration of dynamic attention weights was crucial in enhancing feature representation, leading to more effective learning compared to traditional static attention approaches. Detailed analysis of the learned embeddings further confirmed the advantages of embedding dynamic attention within graph convolutional architectures, significantly improving the capacity to model complex and heterogeneous drug-disease relationships.

A comparative assessment against established approaches, including TL-HGBI, DRRS, DeepDR, NIMGCN, and LAGCN, demonstrated the effectiveness of the proposed model, especially in key evaluation metrics such as predictive precision, retrieval performance, and classification reliability. These findings underscore the importance of the dynamic attention mechanism in enhancing feature discrimination and improving the model's ability to generalize.

In addition to cross-validation results, the practical relevance of the model was showcased through experimental validation on rare diseases, specifically Churg-Strauss Syndrome (EGPA), cystic fibrosis, glioblastoma, and Burkitt lymphoma. Rare diseases were chosen due to their complex biology, limited treatment options, and urgent need for therapeutic innovation. Cystic fibrosis, for instance, was selected because of its severe, progressive nature and the high unmet clinical need despite existing treatments. Through drug repurposing predictions, the model identified promising candidates for these rare diseases, offering a pathway to accelerate therapy development with lower costs and reduced timelines. The findings emphasize that computational drug repurposing, powered by dynamic attention and graph learning, can be a transformative strategy for precision medicine, especially in areas where conventional drug discovery is economically and logistically challenging.

Future directions include enhancing the model with multi-modal biological data, such as gene expression and protein interactions, to improve predictions. Incorporating self-supervised learning and advanced attention schemes may further boost accuracy in drug repurposing. This work offers a reliable and interpretable framework for predicting drug-disease links, supporting progress in drug discovery and precision medicine.

CHAPTER 6

EXPLAINABLE NEURO-SYMBOLIC LEARNING USING MULTI-OMICS DATA FOR DRUG-TARGET-DISEASE PREDICTION IN MULTIPLE CANCER TYPES

6.1 Introduction

In the ever-evolving landscape of precision medicine, the accurate identification of therapeutic targets has emerged as a cornerstone for designing effective and individualized treatment strategies, particularly in oncology. Unlike traditional drug discovery paradigms that primarily emphasize molecular binding affinity or chemical properties, contemporary approaches recognize the need to account for the intricate biological heterogeneity underlying complex diseases. Cancer, for instance, is not a singular condition but a constellation of molecularly diverse subtypes shaped by distinct genetic mutations, transcriptomic alterations, and dysregulated cellular pathways. In this context, therapeutic success depends not only on discovering compounds with high binding affinity, but on precisely mapping druggable targets that are biologically relevant to disease progression and clinical outcome. This paradigm shift has driven increased interest in multi-omics integration and explainable artificial intelligence (AI) frameworks to enable systematic, data-driven identification of actionable gene targets across multiple cancer types. Target identification determines the direction of drug discovery, an incorrect or suboptimal target can result in years of lost research and investment. As studies have shown, targets backed by genetic and molecular evidence significantly increase the likelihood of success in later stages of clinical development [180].

Despite the rising use of computational models in drug discovery pipelines, current methodologies suffer from notable limitations. Traditional machine learning (ML) and deep learning (DL) frameworks are often built on narrow feature spaces, typically centered on molecular or protein interaction data. These models generally overlook the systemic biological complexity encoded in gene expression, mutation profiles, and regulatory networks that influence disease phenotypes. Furthermore, a large fraction of existing models operates as "black boxes," offering little interpretability to clinicians and biomedical researchers. This lack of transparency is particularly concerning when high-stakes decisions must be supported by both biological plausibility and algorithmic robustness.

Recent efforts have shown the potential of integrating gene expression and interaction data to improve target identification. For instance, Dezső and Ceccarelli [181] developed a machine learning model using features derived from proteomics and genomics to prioritize cancer-related targets. Their results underscore the significance of leveraging multi-modal data. Similarly, Bazaga et al. [182] integrated protein-protein interaction (PPI) networks with essentiality and mutation data to identify potential therapeutic targets across nine cancer types, highlighting the importance of disease-specific modelling. While impactful, these approaches often fall short in combining explainability, multi-omics fusion, and downstream drug prioritization in a unified pipeline.

The current research addresses this precise gap by proposing a neuro-symbolic learning framework that combines expert rules, decision trees, and deep learning models to predict therapeutic gene targets from multi-omics datasets, including gene expression, mutation profiles, and topological network features such as degree centrality and PageRank scores. The innovation lies in not only predicting gene targets with high accuracy but also enabling explainable AI through transparent rule-based logic interpretations, enhancing model trustworthiness and biological relevance.

A distinctive aspect of this work is the integration of downstream drug repurposing by predicting drug-target binding affinity (DTBA) using a pre-trained deep learning model. After therapeutic targets are identified across multiple cancer types, known drugs are screened in silico for their interaction potential using molecular SMILES data and protein sequences. This extends the predictive scope beyond binary classification and into actionable therapy suggestions, paving the way for real-world clinical translation.

This framework is grounded in the context of precision oncology, where cancer heterogeneity demands tailored approaches to target discovery. As demonstrated in the Open Targets Platform and The Cancer Genome Atlas (TCGA), high-throughput omics data can uncover cancer-specific molecular aberrations. However, clinical utilization of such data remains suboptimal due to fragmentation across data types and a lack of integration strategies. The proposed framework resolves this by constructing feature-rich datasets that unify expression, mutation, and graph-based representations into a consolidated predictive model.

Inspired by models like OncoRTT [118], which introduced DL-based target prediction per cancer type, the proposed pipeline advances the field in several ways: (i) it introduces a neuro-symbolic learning architecture with interpretable rule-based logic fused with data-driven predictions; (ii) it combines multi-omics features with graph theory to represent complex gene relationships; and (iii) it links therapeutic targets to repurposable drugs using a trained DTBA model, thus completing the cycle from target prediction to actionable pharmacological suggestions.

The methodology is evaluated on datasets spanning four cancer types breast, colon, kidney, and lung, each with curated multi-omics profiles. A weighted ensemble method combines predictions from expert rules, decision tree models (trained from symbolic rules), and deep neural networks. Top therapeutic targets are ranked based on a combined confidence score, and drug candidates are suggested if their predicted interaction score surpasses a biologically validated threshold. The resulting pipeline not only delivers disease-specific, interpretable, and biologically relevant predictions, but also identifies potentially repurposable drugs for each cancer context.

The key contributions of this work are as follows:

1. Developed a novel explainable neuro-symbolic framework for therapeutic target prediction across multiple cancer types, integrating expert rules, symbolic decision trees, and deep learning predictions.
2. Proposed a multi-omics dataset, including expression, mutation, and topological graph features, enhancing both prediction accuracy and biological interpretability.
3. A multimodal pipeline driven by multi-omics data and network topology, yielding ranked, biologically plausible gene targets and high-confidence drug leads, with transparency through rule-based explanations.

In conclusion, this research bridges a critical gap between target identification and drug repurposing by offering an integrated, explainable, and biologically grounded pipeline. It advances the field toward a future where AI-driven insights are not only accurate but also interpretable and actionable, contributing meaningfully to precision oncology and systems-level drug discovery. Future work will involve validating model predictions using patient-derived tumor samples and expanding the framework to incorporate clinical and phenotypic data for even more personalized therapy design.

6.2 Methodology

6.2.1 Problem Definition

Therapeutic Target Identification is modelled as a binary classification problem, where each gene g_i within a cancer-specific dataset is assigned a label $y_i \in \{0,1\}$, indicating whether it is a potential therapeutic target ($y_i = 1$) or not ($y_i = 0$). For each gene g_i, a feature vector is defined as ,

$$\mathrm{x}_i = \left[x_i^{(\mathrm{exp})}, x_i^{(\mathrm{mut})}, x_i^{(\mathrm{topo})}, x_i^{(\mathrm{emb})}\right] \tag{6.1}$$

where:

- $x_i^{(\mathrm{exp})}$ represents gene expression statistics (MAX, AVG, MED, MIN),
- $x_i^{(\mathrm{mut})}$ represents mutation-based features (COUNT, mutation frequency),
- $x_i^{(\mathrm{topo})}$ represents graph-derived features such as degree centrality d_i and PageRank score p_i,
- $x_i^{(emb)}$ represents pre-trained BERT-based embeddings of protein sequences.

Thus, the complete dataset for a cancer type is represented as:

$$\mathcal{D} = \{(\mathrm{x}_i, y_i)\}_{i=1}^{N} \tag{6.2}$$

where N is the number of genes.

To incorporate symbolic knowledge and neural learning, a combined prediction score is defined as:

$$S(g_i) = \alpha R_{\mathrm{exp}}(g_i) + \beta R_{DT}(g_i) + \gamma P_{DL}(g_i) \tag{6.3}$$

where:

- $R_{\mathrm{exp}}(g_i) \in \{0,1\}$ is the expert rule-based score derived from domain-specific symbolic rules.
- $R_{DT}(g_i) \in [0,1]$ is the decision tree prediction, representing the interpretable symbolic learning component.
- $P_{DL}(g_i) \in [0,1]$ is the probability predicted by the deep neural network (DNN).
- α, β, γ are ensemble weights, constrained such that $\alpha + \beta + \gamma = 1$.

A gene g_i is classified as a potential therapeutic target if:

$$\hat{y}_i = \mathbb{I}[S(g_i) \geq \tau] \quad (6.4)$$

where τ is a threshold.

For each predicted target g_i, potential repurposable drugs were identified d_j from a set $\mathcal{D}_{drug}$ using a DrugTarget Binding Affinity (DTBA) model:

$$\hat{I}(g_i, d_j) = f_\theta\left(\text{SMILES}(d_j), \text{Seq}(g_i)\right) \quad (6.5)$$

where:

- $\text{SMILES}(d_j)$ is the chemical structure of the drug encoded via Mol2Vec embeddings,
- $\text{Seq}(g_i)$ is the protein sequence of gene g_i,
- f_θ is the trained DTBA model with parameters θ.

A drug d_j is considered a repurposing candidate if:

$$\hat{I}(g_i, d_j) \geq \kappa \quad (6.6)$$

where " κ" is a threshold based on the KIBA score or binding affinity cut-off.

6.2.2 Data Preprocessing

The effectiveness of any computational drug discovery pipeline heavily depends on the quality and representativeness of the input data. The preprocessing strategy integrates multi-omics data, protein sequence embeddings, network-based features, and drug structure embeddings, ensuring a comprehensive feature space for both therapeutic target identification and drug repurposing. Figure 6.1 illustrates data preprocessing and data integration.

Multi-Omics and Network-Based Graph Feature Extraction

As detailed in Chapter 3, Section 3.3, gene-specific features were derived by integrating both processed multi-omics data and network-based information. From precomputed gene expression profiles, statistical measures like maximum (MAX), average (AVG), median (MED), and minimum (MIN) were extracted, while mutation burden was captured using the mutation count (COUNT) per gene. These features characterize baseline functional activity and genomic instability relevant to cancer progression. Complementing this, gene-specific subgraphs were constructed from the BIOGRID protein–protein interaction (PPI) database by retaining only those genes present in the cancer-specific datasets. Interactions among these genes defined the edges of each subgraph. From these subgraphs, degree centrality, quantifying a gene's direct connectivity, and PageRank score, reflecting its broader influence within the interaction network, were computed. Together, these features integrate molecular activity with systems-level context, supporting the identification of hub genes as potential therapeutic targets.

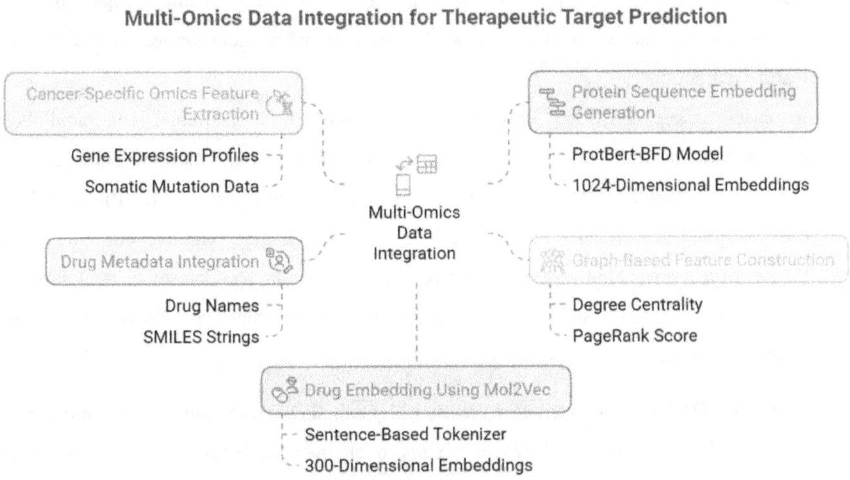

Figure 6.1: Data preprocessing and integration

Protein Sequence Embeddings using ProtBert-BFD

Traditional sequence encoding approaches, such as one-hot encodings or handcrafted amino acid descriptors, fail to capture semantic dependencies within protein sequences. To address this, BERT-based embeddings were generated using the ProtBert-BFD model, which is part of the ProtTrans family of transformer-based models [183]. ProtBert-BFD has been pre-trained on over 2.1 billion protein sequences (BFD-100 dataset), enabling it to learn contextual biochemical patterns from large-scale data. For each gene in the dataset, the amino acid sequence is passed through ProtBert-BFD, and a 1024-dimensional vector representation for each sequence is extracted. These embeddings encode evolutionary information, secondary structure preferences, and functional motifs, which are crucial for differentiating druggable versus non-druggable targets.

Drug Features and Embedding Generation

To facilitate drug repurposing and drug-target interaction prediction, drug-related metadata were systematically integrated and transformed into machine-readable features. The drug information was primarily obtained from the Drug-Gene Interaction Database (DGIdb), which provides curated data linking drugs to their target genes. Each drug entry includes essential attributes such as the drug name, its approval status, unique drug concept identifiers, and experimentally or computationally derived interaction scores (interaction_score). Additionally, SMILES (Simplified Molecular Input Line Entry System) strings, which provide a compact representation of a molecule's structure, were incorporated to enable chemical feature extraction.

In cases where SMILES data were incomplete or unavailable, canonical SMILES representations were generated using a systematic querying pipeline. This pipeline first searches the PubChem database using drug synonyms and chemical identifiers. If PubChem does not yield valid results, the process falls back to ChEMBL searches, either by compound ID or drug name. This ensures that every drug entry in the dataset is associated with a standardized SMILES string, thereby maintaining consistency for downstream molecular feature processing.

Once the SMILES representations were obtained, they were transformed into continuous vector embeddings using Mol2Vec, an approach inspired by natural language processing (NLP) methods. Mol2Vec treats molecular substructures as “words” and entire molecules as “sentences.” The transformation process involves three key stages:

1. Tokenization of SMILES strings - Each SMILES representation is decomposed into substructures using the mol2alt_sentence algorithm with a fixed radius of 2, ensuring that local structural patterns within the molecule are effectively captured.

2. Embedding lookup - A pre-trained Word2Vec model (model_300dim.pkl) is used to map each substructure to a 300-dimensional vector, leveraging the model’s prior knowledge of chemical environments.

3. Vector aggregation - For each drug, the embeddings of its substructures are summed to produce a single 300-dimensional embedding, effectively capturing its global chemical and structural characteristics.

The Mol2Vec embeddings serve as a chemically informed representation of drugs, encoding information about molecular similarity and structural motifs. These embeddings are particularly useful for predicting drug-target binding affinities, as they provide a compact yet expressive feature space that can be combined with protein sequence embeddings to model interactions. By integrating curated drug metadata with chemically enriched Mol2Vec embeddings, the dataset supports explainable drug repurposing by linking therapeutic targets to structurally similar and potentially repurposable compounds.

Feature Integration and Cleaning

For each cancer type, all heterogeneous feature sources multi-omics descriptors (e.g., expression and mutation statistics), protein sequence embeddings, graph-theoretic metrics (Degree Centrality and PageRank Score), and drug metadata are integrated into a single, unified feature matrix. Integration is performed through outer joins on the Gene identifier, ensuring that no candidate gene is discarded due to its absence in any individual data source. To prevent biased exclusion and to maintain a consistent feature space across genes, missing values are systematically imputed with zero, a neutral choice that avoids leakage of label information while enabling downstream learning algorithms to process the complete matrix. The Label column (binary: 0/1), denoting non-target versus putative therapeutic target genes, is preserved to support supervised model training, validation, and evaluation across all subsequent neuro-symbolic and deep learning pipelines.

6.2.3 Model Architecture

This section details the comprehensive methodology adopted for predicting drug-disease associations, emphasizing the architecture of the proposed system and its training procedure. The proposed pipeline tackles two tightly coupled problems:

- Cancer-type-specific therapeutic target identification from multi-omics + network features using an explainable neuro-symbolic learner.
- Drug repurposing for the top-ranked targets by predicting drug-target model and selecting candidates that pass a biologically meaningful threshold.

The architecture integrates domain expert rules, decision-tree (DT) extracted symbolic rules, and a deep neural network (DNN) into a single fusion layer. This design provides (i) interpretability through explicit rules (ii) adaptability through learned neural representations, and (iii) robustness through probabilistic fusion and cross-validated weight tuning.

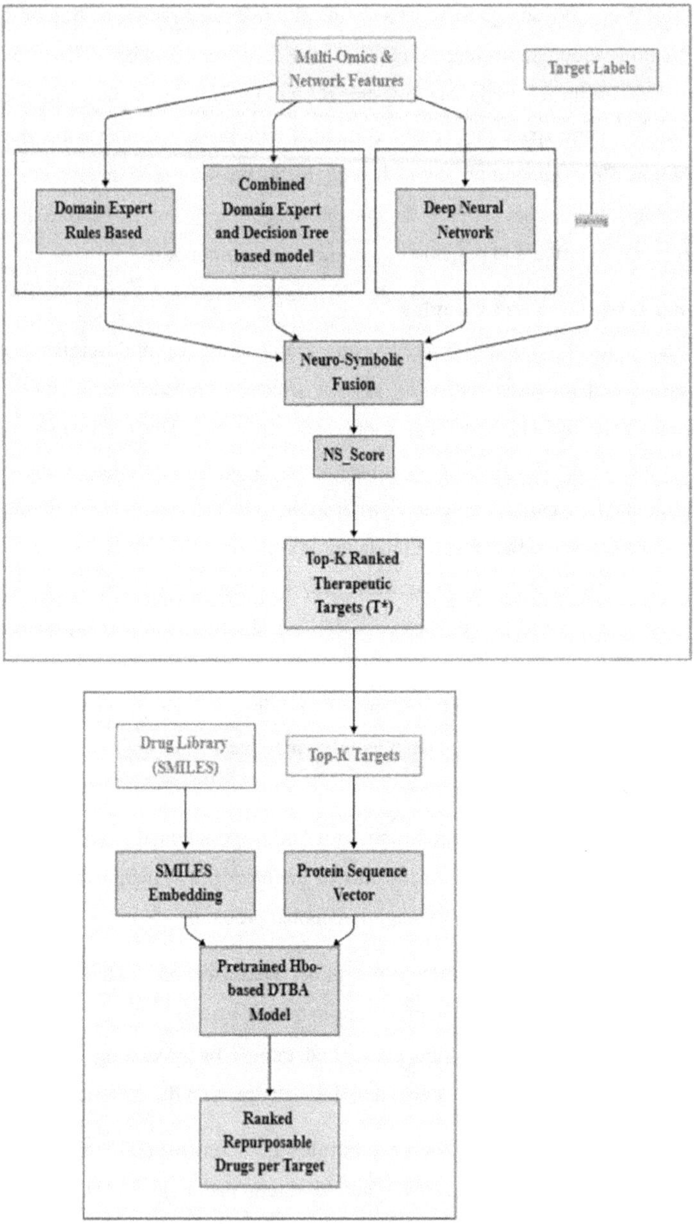

Figure 6.2: Proposed architecture

Algorithm 6.1: Neuro-Symbolic Therapeutic Target Prediction

Input: Multi-omics feature matrix $X \in \mathbb{R}^{n \times m}$ for n genes and m features, Label vector $Y \in \{0,1\}^n$ (target vs. non-target), Expert rule set f_{expert}, Decision tree rule function f_{DT}.

Output: Ranked list of predicted therapeutic targets $\mathcal{T}^*$.

1. Data Preprocessing
   1.1. Integrate multi-omics data (mutation, expression, graph features).
   1.2. Normalize continuous features (e.g., StandardScaler).
   1.3. Construct graph metrics Degree_Centrality and PageRank_Score.

2. Cross-Validation Setup
   2.1. Initialize Stratified K-Fold $\{(X^i_{\text{train}}, X^i_{\text{test}}, Y^i_{\text{train}}, Y^i_{\text{test}})\}_{i=1}^{k}$.
   2.2. Initialize evaluation metrics (Accuracy, F1, AUC, MCC).

3. Model Training & Evaluation (per fold)

   For each fold $i = 1, \dots, k$:
   3.1. Rule-only prediction:

$$\hat{Y}^{(R)} = f_{\text{expert}}\left(X^i_{\text{test}}\right).$$

   Compute metrics $M_i^{(R)}$.
   3.2. DT + Rules (Symbolic Fusion):

$$\hat{Y}^{(S)} = 1\left(\alpha \cdot f_{\text{expert}}\left(X^i_{\text{test}}\right) + (1-\alpha) \cdot f_{\text{DT}}\left(X^i_{\text{test}}\right) \geq 0.5\right).$$

   Compute metrics $M_i^{(S)}$.
   3.3. Deep Learning Model:

   Train f_{DL} on $\left(X^i_{\text{train}}, Y^i_{\text{train}}\right)$.
   Predict $p^{(DL)} = f_{\text{DL}}\left(X^i_{\text{test}}\right)$.

   3.4. Neuro-Symbolic Fusion:

   $S^{(NS)} = \lambda_1 f_{\text{expert}} + \lambda_2 f_{\text{DT}} + \lambda_3 f_{\text{DT}}$.
   Predict $\hat{Y}^{(NS)} = 1\left(S^{(NS)} \geq \tau\right)$.
   Compute metrics $M_i^{(NS)}$.

4. Final Target Ranking
   4.1. Rank genes by $S^{(NS)}$ to form $\mathcal{T}^*$.
   4.2. Select top K targets

End

Algorithm 6.2: Drug Repurposing via HBO-Optimized DTBA
Input: Top gene set $\mathcal{T}^*$, Drug library $\mathcal{D}$ with SMILES strings., Pretrained DTBA model f_{DTBA} (HBO-optimized), Interaction threshold τ_{DtBA}. Output: Ranked list of repurposable drugs per gene. 1. Iterate over Top Genes For each gene $g \in \mathcal{T}^*$: 1.1. Extract protein sequence Seq_g. 2. Drug Interaction Scoring For each drug $d \in \mathcal{D}$: 2.1. Extract chemical structure SMILES $_d$. 2.2. Compute binding affinity: $\hat{s}_{g,d} = f_{\text{DTBA}}(\text{SMILES}_d, \text{Seq}_g)$. 2.3. If $\hat{s}_{g,d} \geq \tau_{\text{DTBA}}$, label (g, d) as repurposable. 3. Drug Ranking 3.1. Sort all $d \in \mathcal{D}$ by $\hat{s}_{g,d}$ for each g. 3.2. Select top M drugs per gene. 4. Output Results 4.1. Return $\mathcal{R} = \{(g, d, \hat{s}_{g,d}): g \in \mathcal{T}^*, d \in \mathcal{D}\}$. End

The final therapeutic target score drives a second module that screens a drug library and outputs repurposable drugs ranked by predicted interaction strength. The complete model architecture and workflow for therapeutic target prediction and identification of top interacting drugs are illustrated in Figure 6.2 and detailed in Algorithms 6.1 and 6.2.

6.2.3.1 Rule-Based Module (Expert Knowledge Engine)

The foundation of the symbolic reasoning component in the hybrid neuro-symbolic framework is a Rule-Based Expert Module a biologically informed decision engine developed independently for each cancer type. These hand-crafted rules leverage domain expertise, published literature, and statistical thresholds to identify potential therapeutic gene targets based on multi-omics and graph-theoretic features. Each rule set integrates overexpression patterns, mutation profiles, and topological prominence in protein-protein interaction (PPI) networks to yield interpretable, high-precision predictions. Each cancer-specific rule module consists of four core classes of criteria:

1. **Oncogenic Overexpression and Network Centrality:** Genes with very high expression values (MAX, AVG) and elevated graph centrality scores (Degree Centrality, PageRank Score) are indicative of oncogenes, often acting as critical drivers in tumorigenesis.
2. **Consistently Elevated Expression Across Patients:** Genes that exhibit uniform high expression across samples (high MIN and MED values), in conjunction with positive mutation evidence and moderate graph activity, reflect stable biomarkers with potential prognostic or therapeutic value.
3. **Hub Regulators with Moderate Expression:** Genes with moderate expression but extremely high topological centrality frequently act as regulatory bottlenecks or signal transduction relays within cellular systems.
4. **Tumor Suppressors with Low Expression but High Network Importance:** Several tumor suppressors display suppressed expression (low MAX), yet maintain high connectivity in molecular interaction graphs. These genes are frequently downregulated or mutated but retain significant biological relevance.

The rules were designed using robust, dataset-specific thresholds derived from a comprehensive analysis of the upper quartile and extreme tail distributions of key multi-omics and graph-based features to ensure high specificity and biological relevance in target selection. Each threshold–feature combination was strategically optimized to capture genes exhibiting high expression levels, frequent mutations, and central network connectivity, as these characteristics indicate functional importance and therapeutic potential. This integrative approach ensures that only biologically meaningful and clinically actionable targets are prioritized. A detailed summary of these expert-curated rules, tailored for each cancer type, is provided in Table 6.1, Expert Knowledge Rules for Target Gene Identification in Different Cancer Types, where each rule outputs a binary decision per gene reflecting compliance with predefined biological criteria.

Table 6.1 : Expert Knowledge Rules for Target Gene Identification in Different Cancer Types

Cancer Type	Rule Conditions	Biological Rationale	Literature Evidence
Breast	MAX > 10000, AVG > 2000, Degree_Centrality > 0.02, PageRank > 0.01	Overexpressed oncogenes like HER2 and MYC are central hubs in signaling networks	[184]
	MIN > 500, MED > 1000, COUNT > 0, PageRank > 0.008	Uniform high expression across samples marks robust biomarkers like ESR1, GATA3	[185, 186]
	AVG > 1000, Degree_Centrality > 0.05, PageRank > 0.015	Hub genes like CDK1 regulate mitosis, crucial in therapy	[187]
Kidney	MAX > 10000, AVG > 2000, Degree_Centrality > 0.015, PageRank > 0.01	Oncogene-like profile; overexpression in genes like VHL, MET, HIF1A	[188]
	MIN > 500, MED > 1000, COUNT > 0, PageRank > 0.008	Robustly upregulated drivers like CA9, EGFR, VEGFA	[189]
	AVG > 1000, Degree_Centrality > 0.03, PageRank > 0.015	Hubs like TP53 are signaling connectors	[190]
	MAX < 800, Degree_Centrality > 0.05, PageRank > 0.02	Silenced tumor suppressors like PBRM1, BAP1 still central in PPI	[189]
Lung	MAX > 10000, AVG > 2000, Degree_Centrality > 0.02, PageRank > 0.01	EGFR, MYC, MET are highly expressed central regulators in NSCLC	[191]
	MIN > 500, MED > 800, COUNT > 0, PageRank > 0.008	Stable expression markers like KRAS, BRAF are upregulated in lung cancer	[192,193]
	AVG > 1000, Degree_Centrality > 0.03, PageRank > 0.015	Hub genes like TP53, ALK drive key interactions	[194,195]
	MAX < 900, Degree_Centrality > 0.035, PageRank > 0.02	Tumor suppressors like KEAP1 and RB1 are downregulated but topologically critical	[196,197]

Formally, this can be described as:

$$\hat{y}^{(R)} = \begin{cases} 1 & \text{if } f_{\text{expert}}(x) = 1 \\ 0 & \text{otherwise} \end{cases} \tag{6.7}$$

Where f_{expert} is the cancer-type-specific Boolean logic composed of the above rules, and x denotes the feature vector for a given gene.

These symbolic decisions act both as stand-alone interpretable models and as foundational priors in the hybrid pipeline. In later stages, these rules are combined with data-driven classifiers such as decision trees and deep neural networks using soft or hard fusion mechanisms, thereby integrating human-curated biological knowledge with automated learning capacity.

6.2.3.2 Symbolic Module: Decision Tree + Expert Rule Fusion

The symbolic module forms the second layer of the proposed neuro-symbolic architecture, designed to integrate interpretable machine learning with domain-specific biological knowledge. This layer aims to enhance prediction accuracy while preserving interpretability through rule-based reasoning. The module operates in two complementary phases: (1) Extraction of symbolic rules from a decision tree classifier, and (2) Fusion of these data-driven symbolic rules with expert-curated rules tailored for each cancer type.

Decision Tree Rule Extraction

For each cancer type, a Decision Tree (DT) classifier is trained using the same unified feature matrix derived from pre-processed features. The DT is chosen due to its inherent interpretability each path from root to leaf can be translated into a human-readable *if-then* rule. After training, the paths of the decision tree are programmatically extracted and converted into executable Python functions. These automatically generated symbolic rules are then compiled into separate modules per cancer and dynamically imported at runtime. This setup ensures scalability and modularity for future cancer types.

Expert Rule Module

In parallel, domain knowledge is encoded into hand-crafted expert rules. These rules are constructed using thresholds on gene expression metrics (MAX, AVG, MED, MIN, COUNT) and network topology features (Degree_Centrality, PageRank_Score). A unique rule function is defined for each cancer type, reflecting its distinct biological characteristics (e.g., overexpression patterns, mutation burden, or centrality in protein interaction networks). The rationale and thresholds for these rules are grounded in peer-reviewed biomedical literature.

Fusion Strategy

To leverage both data-driven symbolic reasoning and expert domain knowledge, the predictions from the expert rule engine $\left(\hat{y}^{(R)}\right)$ and the decision tree classifier $\left(\hat{y}^{(DT)}\right)$ are combined through a probabilistic fusion mechanism defined as:

$$s^{(S)} = \alpha \cdot \hat{y}^{(R)} + (1 - \alpha) \cdot \hat{y}^{(DT)} \tag{6.8}$$

$$\hat{y}^{(S)} = \begin{cases} 1 & \text{if } s^{(S)} \geq \tau \\ 0 & \text{otherwise} \end{cases} \tag{6.9}$$

Where:

- $\alpha \in [0,1]$ is a fusion weight hyperparameter optimized via cross-validation,
- τ is the decision threshold, typically set to 0.5 .

The fusion score $s^{(S)}$ reflects a soft combination of the expert logic and symbolic decision tree reasoning. This hybrid mechanism enhances generalizability while retaining interpretability, as both contributing components are rule-based.

6.2.3.3 Deep Learning Module and Neuro-Symbolic Fusion

To enhance the model's representational capacity and exploit non-linear interactions among features, the third module in the proposed framework incorporates a deep neural network (DNN). This module is trained on the same unified and normalized feature matrix used by the symbolic models. It serves as a high-capacity learner that complements the interpretability of rule-based and symbolic approaches. The network architecture consists of two fully connected hidden layers. Each layer is followed by an activation function either sigmoid or tanh selected through hyperparameter optimization. L2 regularization is applied to both kernel weights and biases to mitigate overfitting. The output layer uses a sigmoid activation function to produce a probability score $p^{(DL)} \in [0,1]$, representing the likelihood of a gene being a therapeutic target:

The network learns complex, high-dimensional representations that may be elusive to linear or rule-based models, enabling improved sensitivity to latent gene-drug-cancer interactions.

Hyperparameters governing the architecture, activation functions, and regularization strengths were optimized using the Keras Tuner with Bayesian optimization to maximize classification metrics such as F1-score, AUC, and Matthews Correlation Coefficient (MCC). The best-performing configuration is summarized in Table 6.2. The model was trained using binary cross-entropy loss and the Adam optimizer, with early stopping based on validation performance.

Table 6.2: Optimized Hyperparameters of Deep Neural Network

Hyperparameter	**Value**
Units in Layer 1	256
Activation (Layer 1)	Sigmoid
Units in Layer 2	48
Activation (Layer 2)	Sigmoid
L2 Kernel Regularization	0.001698
L2 Bias Regularization	0.002484
Learning Rate	0.0006177

Neuro-Symbolic Fusion

To integrate the complementary strengths of the expert-driven rule module, symbolic decision tree model, and the deep neural network, a neuro-symbolic fusion strategy is adopted. This approach combines predictions from all three modules using a weighted linear combination to produce a final decision score $S^{(NS)}$

$$S^{(NS)} = \lambda_1 \cdot \hat{y}^{(R)} + \lambda_2 \cdot \hat{y}^{(DT)} + \lambda_3 \cdot p^{(DL)} \quad (6.10)$$

$$\hat{y}^{(NS)} = \begin{cases} 1 & \text{if } S^{(NS)} \geq \tau \\ 0 & \text{otherwise} \end{cases} \quad (6.11)$$

Where:

- $\hat{y}^{(R)} \in \{0,1\}$ is the prediction from the rule-based expert module,

- $\hat{y}^{(DT)} \in \{0,1\}$ is the prediction from the decision tree classifier,
- $p^{(DL)} \in [0,1]$ is the probability from the DNN,
- $\lambda_1 + \lambda_2 + \lambda_3 = 1$, with $\lambda_i \geq 0$,
- $\tau \in [0,1]$ is the decision threshold.

These weights λ_i and threshold τ are tuned to maximize validation AUC, F1-score, and MCC.

6.2.3.4 Drug Repurposing Module

The final stage of the proposed pipeline focuses on the identification of potential repurposed drugs for cancer-specific therapeutic targets. This is accomplished by leveraging the outputs from the previously developed neuro-symbolic model, which provides a ranked list of gene candidates most likely to serve as valid therapeutic targets for each cancer type.

To perform drug repurposing, the predicted target genes are first mapped to their corresponding protein sequences. These sequences, along with candidate drug compounds, are then supplied to the HBO-optimized Drug-Target Binding Affinity (DTBA) prediction model developed as part of the first research objective, detailed in Chapter 4 (section 4.1). This model evaluates the likelihood of interaction between target proteins and candidate drugs based on their molecular representations and predicted binding affinities.

The candidate drugs are sourced from the BioGRID 4.4.242 dataset, which provides a comprehensive collection of curated protein-protein and protein-drug interactions. The BioGRID release used was compiled on January 25, 2025, and includes all curated interaction data available up to that date. This release is chosen for its inclusion of FDA-approved drugs, ensuring clinical relevance and translational potential of the repurposing predictions.

This integrative approach enables the identification of high-confidence drug candidates that can be repurposed for targeted therapy against specific cancers. It combines symbolic reasoning, deep learning, and biological interaction networks to ensure both interpretability and predictive accuracy in repurposing decisions.

6.3 Evaluation Metrics

To rigorously assess the performance of the proposed multi-module drug-target prediction framework across diverse cancer types, a comprehensive suite of evaluation metrics were employed. These metrics are designed to capture various aspects of model behavior, including correctness, robustness, class balance handling, and discrimination capability. The following metrics are used throughout the experiments like accuracy, precision, recall, specificity, F1-score, area under the ROC curve (AUC), and Matthews correlation coefficient (MCC). Detailed definitions and in-depth interpretation of Accuracy, F1-Score, AUC, and Specificity, refer to chapter 5(section 5.3). An elaboration of the remaining metrics is provided below.

Precision

Precision quantifies the proportion of true positive predictions among all positive predictions made by the model. It is particularly important in biomedical applications such as drug-target identification, where false positives can lead to costly or harmful downstream experiments. High precision indicates a low false-positive rate, reflecting the model's ability to avoid incorrectly labeling non-target genes as targets.

$$\text{Precision} = \frac{TP}{TP+FP} \tag{6.12}$$

Matthews Correlation Coefficient (MCC)

The Matthews Correlation Coefficient is a robust measure that account for true and false positives and negatives, and is generally regarded as a balanced evaluation metric, especially useful when dealing with imbalanced datasets.

$$\text{MCC} = \frac{TP \cdot TN - FP \cdot FN}{\sqrt{(TP+FP)(TP+FN)(TN+F\ )(TN+FN)}} \tag{6.13}$$

MCC returns a value between -1 and 1 :

- A value of 1 indicates perfect prediction
- 0 indicates random prediction,
- -1 indicates total disagreement between prediction and observation.

6.4 Results and Analysis

This section presents a comprehensive comparative analysis of the predictive performance of the three proposed modules, Rule-Based Only, Symbolic Fusion (Decision Tree + Expert Rules), and Neuro-Symbolic Model (Deep Neural Network + Symbolic Fusion) , across five major cancer types: Breast, Colon, Kidney, Liver, and Lung. The evaluation is conducted using seven widely accepted classification metrics: Accuracy, Precision, Recall, Specificity,

Table 6.3: Performance Comparison Across Models and Cancer Types

Metric	Cancer Type	Rule-Based Only	Decision Tree + Rules (Combined)	Neural Net + DT + Domain Rules (Neuro-Symbolic)
Accuracy	Breast	0.5743	0.8895	**0.8964**
	Bladder	0.5315	0.7926	**0.8214**
	Lung	0.5774	0.8803	**0.8839**
	Kidney	0.5235	0.8377	**0.8413**
Precision	Breast	0.3	0.8848	**0.9**
	Bladder	0.6635	0.7513	**0.795**
	Lung	0.7333	0.8761	**0.8826**
	Kidney	0.4	0.7965	**0.8023**
Recall	Breast	0.032	**0.856**	**0.856**
	Bladder	0.1831	**0.9049**	0.8889
	Lung	0.048	**0.848**	**0.848**
	Kidney	0.0225	**0.896**	**0.896**
Specificity	Breast	**0.9879**	0.915	0.9271
	Bladder	0.913	0.6696	**0.7478**
	Lung	**0.9935**	0.9054	0.9119
	Kidney	**0.9929**	0.7837	0.7909
F1-score	Breast	0.0577	0.8698	**0.877**
	Bladder	0.282	0.8206	**0.839**
	Lung	0.089	0.8603	**0.8638**
	Kidney	0.0424	0.8416	**0.8445**
AUC	Breast	0.5099	0.8855	**0.9357**
	Bladder	0.5481	0.7872	**0.8786**
	Lung	0.5208	0.8767	**0.9125**
	Kidney	0.5077	0.8399	**0.8816**
MCC	Breast	0.0359	0.7746	**0.7889**
	Bladder	0.1282	0.5954	**0.6458**
	Lung	0.1247	0.758	**0.7647**
	Kidney	0.0416	0.6851	**0.6922**

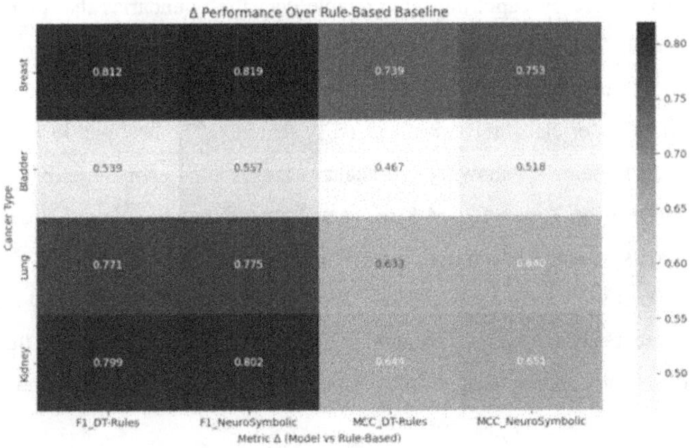

Figure 6.3: Performance Improvement (Δ) Over Rule-Based Baseline Across Cancer Types

F1-Score, AUC, and Matthews Correlation Coefficient (MCC), ensuring a thorough assessment of each model's behavior. As shown in Table 6.3, the performance improves consistently with increasing model complexity, clearly demonstrating the incremental value of integrating symbolic reasoning and neural learning mechanisms over traditional expert rule-based approaches in enhancing predictive reliability and generalization.. Key findings include:

- The Rule-Based Model, while interpretable and high in specificity, suffers from extremely low recall and F1-scores across all cancer types, indicating a high false-negative rate and limited generalization.
- The Symbolic Fusion Model, combining decision tree logic with domain rules, shows a substantial gain in all metrics, especially recall and F1-score, suggesting improved identification of target genes without sacrificing interpretability.
- The Neuro-Symbolic Model achieves the best trade-off between precision and recall, yielding the highest scores in terms of Accuracy, F1-Score, AUC, and MCC across most cancer types. This demonstrates the benefit of integrating deep feature learning with rule-based inference.

Overall, these results validate the effectiveness of the proposed hierarchical hybrid learning strategy in improving prediction performance across multiple metrics. The introduction of the symbolic reasoning layer, integrating decision trees and expert-derived rules, notably enhances recall and F1-score by capturing interpretable decision boundaries that pure neural models often overlook. The final neuro-symbolic fusion combining deep neural representations with symbolic logic and domain knowledge further improves AUC and MCC values, key indicators of robustness under class imbalance and noisy features. The heatmap in Figure 6.3 visually demonstrates these gains, showing consistent increases in F1-score and MCC achieved by the Symbolic (Decision Tree + Expert Rules) and Neuro-Symbolic (Neural Net + DT + Domain Rules) models over the baseline rule-based approach across cancer types. The comparative performance of the baseline model[182], OncoRTT[118], and the proposed integrated model across different cancer types is illustrated in Figure 6.4. The results indicate that the integrated model consistently achieves higher AUC values for breast, bladder, lung, and kidney cancers

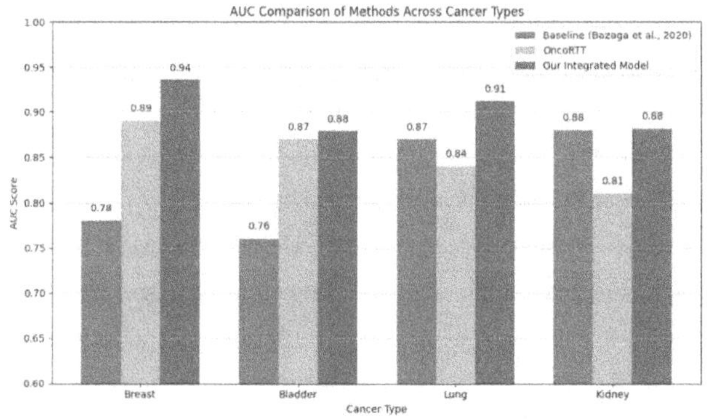

Figure 6.4: AUC comparison of baseline, OncoRTT, and the integrated model across multiple cancer types.

6.4.1 Experimental validation

To rigorously assess the biological and clinical relevance of the predicted therapeutic targets, a multi-tiered validation framework was employed, integrating expression profiling, survival analysis, and druggability assessment. Expression validation was conducted using TNMplot, which evaluates differential gene expression between tumor and normal tissues. Genes were considered overexpressed in tumor tissues if the mean fold change exceeded 2 ($log_2FC > 1$) and the corresponding p-value was < 0.001, indicating statistically significant upregulation. Prognostic significance was assessed via Kaplan-Meier Plotter (KMPlot), where a gene was deemed clinically relevant if the hazard ratio (HR) significantly deviated from 1, either protective (HR < 1) or risk-associated (HR > 1), with a log-rank p-value < 0.05. Only targets satisfying either strong overexpression criteria or exhibiting statistically significant survival impact were retained for further analysis.

Druggability assessment was performed using curated databases, including DGIdb, Open Targets, and DrugBank, which were cross-referenced with peer-reviewed literature to confirm the feasibility of pharmacological modulation. For each validated target, potential interacting drugs were identified using the Drug Target Binding Affinity (DTBA) model proposed in Chapter 4 and shortlisted based on high predicted binding scores. These drug target pairs were further supported by existing experimental or clinical evidence, enhancing translational potential. In addition, drug-disease associations predicted by the neuro-symbolic framework for multiple cancer types were systematically validated using the above resources, providing candidate suggestions for future research. These validated associations represent novel opportunities for drug repurposing and can guide experimental studies or early-stage clinical investigations. For each target gene, the top two FDA-approved drugs with the highest predicted binding affinity were identified and recommended as prioritized candidates for translational follow-up.

This multi-parameter validation strategy, combining statistical thresholds ($\log_2 FC > 1$, $p < 0.001$, $HR \neq 1$ with $p < 0.05$), expression profiling, clinical survival relevance, and drug-target binding scores, ensures that the identified candidates are computationally robust, biologically meaningful, and translationally actionable. This approach lays a strong foundation for future experimental validation and precision oncology applications.

This work focused on breast, lung, bladder, and kidney cancers, representing a spectrum of highly prevalent malignancies with distinct etiological drivers and therapeutic challenges. These cancers were prioritized based on three key considerations:

1. **Epidemiological significance** - Each cancer type ranks among the leading causes of cancer incidence and mortality globally, accounting for a substantial proportion of the cancer burden.

2. **Therapeutic gaps** - Despite available treatment regimens, these cancers exhibit resistance to standard therapies, limited targeted options, or poor long-term survival outcomes.

3. **Biological diversity** - The selected cancers collectively represent hormone-driven malignancies (breast), environmentally associated tumours (lung, bladder), and metabolically linked cancers (liver), allowing us to evaluate the generalizability of the proposed framework across distinct pathophysiological contexts.

Following multi-tier validation, the predicted therapeutic targets and their top repurposable FDA-approved drugs were compiled for each cancer type. For each cancer type, targets were validated based on tumor-specific overexpression, prognostic significance, and druggability, and the highest-affinity drugs were identified using the DTBA model. The following subsections describe the validation outcomes for each cancer.

6.4.1.1 Breast Cancer

Breast cancer represents the most common malignancy among women worldwide and remains a leading cause of cancer-related mortality despite significant advances in screening, molecular subtyping, and targeted therapeutics. According to global cancer statistics, breast cancer accounts for more than 2.3 million new cases annually, contributing to nearly 700,000 deaths[198]. Although improvements in early detection and the introduction of endocrine therapy, HER2-directed monoclonal antibodies, and CDK4/6 inhibitors have transformed patient outcomes, the disease continues to pose major clinical challenges.

Tumor heterogeneity, the emergence of resistance to standard therapies, and the lack of effective treatments for aggressive subtypes such as triple-negative breast cancer (TNBC) underscore the urgent need for novel therapeutic strategies.

Within this context, breast cancer was selected as a priority case study owing to its high prevalence, complex biology, and pressing therapeutic gaps. The proposed neuro-symbolic framework identified a set of candidate therapeutic targets that were subsequently subjected to the multi-tier validation pipeline. Expression profiling using TNMplot confirmed that several genes were significantly upregulated in tumor tissues compared to matched normal counterparts, with stringent thresholds applied ($\log_2 FC > 1$, $p < 0.001$). This provided strong evidence of tumor-specific dysregulation, reinforcing the biological relevance of the identified candidates.

To complement expression analysis, prognostic evaluation was performed using Kaplan-Meier Plotter (KMPlot), which stratified breast cancer patients into high- and low-expression groups.

Genes demonstrating a significant deviation in hazard ratio (HR < 1 for protective or HR > 1 for risk-associated, log-rank $p < 0.05$) were classified as clinically meaningful.

Table 6.4: Predicted therapeutic targets for breast cancer with multi-tier validation.

Target	Overexpressed	Prognostic	PPI / Druggable Context	Literature Evidence	Candidate type
RUVBL1	Yes ($log_2FC = 0.95$; $p = 6.74e-05$)	High expression → Poor survival (HR = 1.35; p = 6.9e-09)	Chromatin remodeling complexes; druggable interactor context	[199], [200]	Validated therapeutic target
IL13RA1	Mild ($log_2FC \approx 0.16$; $p = 8.77e-04$)	High expression → Better survival (HR = 0.89; p = 0.0175)	Cytokine receptor (IL-13/IL-4); JAK/STAT signaling	[201], [202]	Established prognostic & therapeutic target
PCNA	Yes ($log_2FC \approx 1.05$; $p = 1.72e-09$)	High expression → Poor survival (HR = 1.52; p = 3.2e-16)	DNA replication marker; druggable via replication-targeting agents	[203]	Clinically actionable target
LIMK2	Yes ($log_2FC = 0.76$; $p = 1.85e-06$)	Not significant (HR = 1.04; p = 0.396)	Kinase; druggable via LIMK inhibitors	[204], [205]	Experimental therapeutic candidate
CDK7	Yes ($log_2FC = 0.43$; $p = 8.86e-03$)	Not significant (HR = 1.10; p = 0.064)	CDK family; several inhibitors in trials	[206], [207]	Potential context-specific prognostic marker

This ensured that only those targets with a measurable impact on patient survival were advanced for further consideration. Such integration of transcriptomic and survival evidence strengthens the clinical interpretability of the findings, making them more actionable for translational oncology. In the final stage, druggability assessment was performed using curated resources (DGIdb, Open Targets, and DrugBank), which confirmed the feasibility of pharmacological modulation for the majority of validated targets.

Importantly, the Drug Target Binding Affinity (DTBA) model predicted strong interactions between these targets and FDA-approved compounds, highlighting their potential for rapid repurposing. Table 6.4 presents the predicted therapeutic targets and their validation results across the three criteria tumor-specific expression, prognostic significance, and druggability. Table 6.5 further summarizes the top FDA-approved drugs prioritized by high binding affinity scores, representing the most promising candidates for translational follow-up. Taken together, these results demonstrate that the proposed neuro-symbolic framework not only identifies biologically robust and clinically relevant targets in breast cancer but also couples them with actionable drug repurposing opportunities. By bridging expression, survival, and drug-target interaction data, this validation pipeline provides a comprehensive foundation for future pre-clinical investigations and precision oncology applications in breast cancer.

Table 6.5: Top predicted repurposable drugs for validated breast cancer targets.

Target gene	**Predicted drugs**	**Literature evidence**
RUVBL1	Sorafenib, Rottlerin	[207,208]
IL13RA1	Tralokinumab, Lebrikizumab	[209,210]
PCNA	Hypericin, Palbociclib	[211]
LIMK2	Fasudil	[212]
CDK7	Samuraciclib	[213,214]

6.4.1.2 Bladder cancer

Bladder cancer represents a major global health burden, with its incidence steadily increasing, particularly among aging populations and in regions with elevated exposure to tobacco smoke, industrial chemicals, and environmental carcinogens such as aromatic amines. It ranks among the top ten most frequently diagnosed cancers worldwide and remains the most prevalent malignancy of the urinary tract. Despite advancements in surgical and chemotherapeutic strategies, including transurethral resection of bladder tumors (TURBT), intravesical Bacillus Calmette-Guérin (BCG) immunotherapy, and platinum-based systemic regimens, clinical management of bladder cancer continues to be challenging due to its high recurrence rate and frequent progression to muscle-invasive bladder cancer (MIBC). Approximately 50–70% of patients experience disease relapse within five years, and many progress to invasive or metastatic stages, where prognosis remains poor and therapeutic options are limited.

In recent years, immunotherapeutic approaches-particularly immune checkpoint inhibitors (ICIs) targeting PD-1, PD-L1, and CTLA-4 pathways-have transformed the therapeutic landscape of advanced bladder cancer. While these agents, such as pembrolizumab and atezolizumab, have shown encouraging results in subsets of patients, the overall response rates remain modest, typically benefiting fewer than one-third of treated individuals. This highlights the pressing need to identify novel molecular targets and to develop predictive biomarkers that can improve patient stratification and therapeutic efficacy. Given these unmet needs, bladder cancer emerges as an ideal candidate for drug repurposing strategies, wherein existing FDA-approved drugs with established safety profiles are redirected toward new oncological indications. Such approaches offer a time- and cost-efficient route to therapeutic innovation by leveraging known pharmacodynamics and clinical data.In the present study, a neuro-symbolic computational framework was employed to systematically identify bladder cancer-specific therapeutic targets. The framework integrated knowledge-driven reasoning with machine learning-based inference to pinpoint candidate genes implicated in tumorigenesis and disease progression. To ensure biological and clinical validity, the identified targets underwent multi-tier validation. Expression analysis using TNMplot revealed that several candidate genes were significantly overexpressed in tumor tissues relative to normal bladder samples, with stringent statistical thresholds ($\log_2$ fold change > 1; $p < 0.001$). Prognostic assessment via Kaplan-Meier Plotter (KMPlot) demonstrated that a subset of these targets significantly influenced overall survival, as evidenced by hazard ratios deviating substantially from unity, indicating either adverse or protective prognostic significance. Subsequent druggability evaluation using curated and comprehensive databases such as DGIdb, Open Targets, and DrugBank, supplemented by extensive manual literature cross-validation, confirmed both the pharmacological relevance and clinical feasibility of the identified targets. Each shortlisted gene demonstrated established or predicted drug–target interactions, reinforcing their potential for therapeutic modulation. Table 6.6 presents the final panel of bladder cancer-specific therapeutic targets that fulfilled all validation benchmarks, integrating tumor-specific expression, prognostic association, and druggability evidence. .

Table 6.6: Predicted therapeutic targets for bladder cancer with validation

Gene	**Overexpressed**	**Prognostic**	**Druggable**	**Literature Evidence**	**Candidate Type**
GOLPH3	Yes ($log_2FC \approx 2.1$, p = 9.44e-05)	No (KMPlot p = 0.7; HR not significant)	Druggable, Golgi protein, involved in mTOR signaling	[215,216]	Experimental therapeutic candidate
TGFB3	No (downregulated in tumor)	Yes (p = 0.008, high expression → worse survival)	druggable	[217,218]	Established prognostic & therapeutic target
HMGB1	Yes (Mean FC ≈ 1.22; Tumor > Normal in 100% samples at Min/Q1)	Yes - High expression correlates with worse prognosis (p = 0.018)	Indirectly druggable (via HMGB1 inhibitors or RAGE/TLR4 blockade)	[219,220]	Clinically actionable target
GNAI3	Yes (Fold change >1.5, p = 1.62e-03)	Yes (High expression linked to worse survival, p = 0.031)	druggable	[221]	Established prognostic & therapeutic target
MTA1	Yes (overexpressed in tumor, p = 0.00183, fold change > 1)	No (p = 0.63, not statistically significant)	Indirectly (via chromatin remodeling and metastasis-pathways)	[222]	prognostic marker

Thereafter, the Drug-Target Binding Affinity (DTBA) model was implemented to predict, quantify, and rank FDA-approved drugs by their binding affinities, identifying the most promising candidates for repurposing and translational follow-up studiesTable 6.7 presents the top-scoring drugs for each validated target, with particular emphasis on compounds originally developed for other cancer types but showing strong binding predictions in bladder cancer. These include chemotherapeutics, kinase inhibitors, and immune-modulating agents, many of which already have established safety profiles, thereby lowering the barrier to clinical translation.

Table 6.7: Top predicted drugs predicted for validated bladder cancer targets

Gene	Interacting Drug(s)	Literature-based evidence
GOLPH3	Bromocriptine, sulforaphane, Glycyrrhizin	[223,224]
TGFB3	Galunisertib,Fresolimumab	[225,226]
HMGB1	Dexamethasone, Sulforaphane	[227]
GNAI3	Pitavastatin	[228]
MTA1	Argatroban, Demeclocycline	[229]

Collectively, these findings provide a rational foundation for repositioning FDA-approved agents as therapeutic candidates in bladder cancer. The multi-tier validation approach ensures that the shortlisted drug-gene associations are statistically robust, clinically meaningful, and translationally feasible. These results represent actionable opportunities for pre-clinical and clinical follow-up, addressing a critical unmet need in the management of bladder cancer.

6.4.1.3 Lung cancer

Lung cancer is the leading cause of cancer-related mortality globally, accounting for approximately 1.8 million deaths annually and representing a major global health burden. It is broadly classified into non-small cell lung cancer (NSCLC), which constitutes nearly 85% of cases, and small cell lung cancer (SCLC), which is less common but more aggressive. Despite advances in screening and early detection, the majority of patients are diagnosed at advanced stages, where curative options are limited.

Table 6.8: Predicted therapeutic targets for lung cancer with validation

Gene	Overexpressed	Prognostic	Druggable	Literature Evidence	Candidate Type or Can Be Target
CDK2	Yes (Fold change = 5.89; p = 1.56e-106)	Yes (HR = 0.82, 95% CI: 0.73-0.92; p = 0.001)	Yes (well-known kinase target)	[230,231]	Prognostic biomarker (high expression but associated with better survival)
ONECUT2	No (Fold change < 1; p = 0.0702)	Yes (HR = 1.25, 95% CI: 1.11-1.41; p = 0.00021)	Potentially (G-protein family)	[232,233]	Prognostic biomarker (less likely therapeutic target due to low expression)
HIST1H2BL	Yes (Fold change = 1.43; p = 2.34e-04)	Yes (HR = 1.18, 95% CI: 1.05-1.33; p = 0.0066)	Unlikely (Histone protein family)	[234]	Prognostic biomarker (less likely therapeutic target)
RPS6KA2	Yes (Fold change = 1.88; p = 3.74e-43)	No (HR = 0.93, 95% CI: 0.82-1.04; p = 0.21)	Yes (RSK family kinase)	[235]	Overexpressed, non-prognostic, druggable; potential biomarker or target if contextually validated
KRAS	No (Fold change < 1; p = 1.76e-07)	Yes (HR = 0.85, 95% CI: 0.76-0.96; p = 0.0079)	Yes (well-known oncogene, targeted in multiple cancers)	[236]	Prognostic biomarker (less likely therapeutic target in low-expression context)

Standard treatment approaches, including chemotherapy, radiotherapy, and targeted therapies, have improved survival outcomes over the past two decades; however, drug resistance and disease recurrence remain pervasive challenges..

The advent of molecularly targeted therapies has transformed the treatment landscape for subsets of NSCLC, particularly with the development of inhibitors against EGFR, ALK, and ROS1 alterations. More recently, KRAS G12C inhibitors and immune checkpoint inhibitors (such as PD-1/PD-L1 and CTLA-4 antibodies) have expanded the therapeutic arsenal. Nevertheless, only a fraction of patients derive long-term benefit from these therapies, largely due to intratumoral heterogeneity, adaptive signaling mechanisms, and the rapid emergence of resistance mutations. These limitations underscore the urgent need for identifying novel therapeutic targets and drug repurposing opportunities that can complement or overcome current treatment gaps. Within this study, the proposed neuro-symbolic framework was applied to identify and validate putative therapeutic targets for lung cancer using a multi-tiered strategy. Expression profiling with TNMplot revealed a subset of genes that were consistently overexpressed in tumor tissues relative to normal controls, with fold change thresholds ($log_2FC > 1$, $p < 0.001$) ensuring statistical rigor. Prognostic assessment through Kaplan-Meier survival analysis further demonstrated that several of these targets were significantly correlated with patient outcomes, with hazard ratios deviating from unity ($HR < 1$ for protective, $HR > 1$ for risk-associated) and log-rank p-values < 0.05.

Table 6.9: Top predicted drugs predicted for validating lung cancer targets

Gene	Interacting Drug(s)	Literature-based evidence
CDK2	Imatinib, Paclitaxel	[237–239]
ONECUT2	Trichostatin A (TSA), Vorinostat (SAHA), Romidepsin	No evidence
HIST1H2BL	Azacitidine, Tazemetostat	[240–242]
RPS6KA2	Trametinib	[243,24b4]
KRAS	Sotorasib, Adagrasib	[244–246]

Subsequent druggability analysis, performed using DGIdb, Open Targets, and DrugBank, identified potential pharmacological modulators for these validated targets. Candidate drug-target interactions were cross-validated with the Drug Target Binding Affinity (DTBA) model, and the top two FDA-approved drugs for each target were prioritized based on high predicted binding scores. These findings not only support the translational potential of the proposed framework but also highlight clinically actionable opportunities for drug repurposing in lung cancer.

Table 6.8 presents the predicted therapeutic targets validated for tumor-specific expression, prognostic significance, and druggability, while Table 6.9 summarizes the top FDA-approved drugs predicted for these targets. Collectively, these results demonstrate how computational validation can bridge the gap between molecular profiling and therapeutic application, offering promising candidates for future experimental and clinical investigation in lung cancer

6.4.1.4 Kidney cancer

Kidney cancer, specifically renal cell carcinoma (RCC), stands as one of the most significant contributors to the global cancer burden, accounting for approximately 2-3% of all malignancies worldwide. Over the past few decades, the incidence of RCC has shown a steady increase, primarily driven by advances in imaging technology and improvements in early detection methods. Despite these strides in diagnostic capabilities, a significant proportion of RCC patients continue to present with advanced or metastatic disease, where treatment options remain limited and outcomes are poor. Clear cell RCC (ccRCC) is the predominant histological subtype, accounting for the majority of RCC cases, and is characterized by frequent genetic alterations such as mutations in the VHL (Von Hippel-Lindau) gene. These mutations result in the dysregulation of the hypoxia-inducible factor (HIF) pathway, which plays a crucial role in regulating cellular responses to hypoxia and contributes to the malignant behavior of the tumor. As a result, ccRCC tumors are often highly vascularized, which makes them responsive to anti-angiogenic therapies targeting vascular endothelial growth factor (VEGF) and its receptors (VEGFR).

Despite advancements in surgical techniques and the introduction of systemic therapies, kidney cancer remains a major clinical challenge, particularly in the advanced stages of the disease. The therapeutic landscape for RCC has evolved in recent years with the advent of immune checkpoint inhibitors, which have shown promise in enhancing the immune system's ability to

Table 6.10: Predicted therapeutic targets for kidney cancer with validation

Gene	Overexpressed	Prognostic	Druggable	Literature Evidence	Candidate Type or Can Be Target
FOSL1	Yes (Fold change = 1.15; p = 0.0188)	Yes (p = 0.012; high expression linked to worse survival)	Potentially (Transcription factor; indirect targeting possible)	[247]	Prognostic biomarker and potential target (needs functional validation)
LRP2	No (Fold change = 0.38; p = 4.01e-56)	Yes (p < 0.0001)	Yes (LRP2 is a receptor protein; targetable in other diseases)	[248]	Prognostic biomarker (less likely therapeutic target due to low expression)
TYROBP	Yes (Fold change = 4.30; p = 4e-74)	Yes (KMPlot p = 0.017; high expression impacts survival)	Potentially (immune signaling adapter, associated with ITAM)	[249]	Prognostic biomarker and potential immunotherapy target
LIF	No (Fold change = 1.15; p = 0.158)	Yes (p = 0.00073)	Yes (well-known oncogene, targeted in multiple cancers)	[250]	Prognostic biomarker and validated therapeutic target in subsets (e.g., KRAS G12C inhibitors)
RARB	No (Fold change ≈ 1; p = 0.987)	Yes (p < 0.0001 in KMplot)	Yes (Retinoic acid receptor family; nuclear receptor class)	[251]	Prognostic biomarker (less likely therapeutic target due to lack of differential expression)

recognize and target tumor cells. Anti-angiogenic agents that block VEGF/VEGFR signaling pathways have also demonstrated clinical benefit in extending patient survival.

Table 6.11: Top predicted drugs predicted for validating kidney cancer targets

Gene	Interacting Drug(s)	Literature-based evidence
FOSL1	Bosutinib, Levetiracetam	[252,253]
LRP2	Gentamicin, Polymyxin B	[254,255]
TYROBP	Varenicline, Rapamycin, Tacrolimus	[256,257]
LIF	Tocilizumab	[258]
RARB	Adapalene, Tazarotene	[259–261]

Furthermore, combination therapies involving immunotherapy and tyrosine kinase inhibitors (TKIs) are being explored to improve patient outcomes. While these treatments have led to improvements in overall survival, they are not curative, and resistance to these therapies often develops over time. As a result, many patients experience disease progression and limited long-term survival, highlighting the urgent need for novel therapeutic strategies that can overcome these challenges.In light of these issues, the identification of new molecular targets for kidney cancer treatment has become a critical area of research. The current study applied a neuro-symbolic framework to analyze kidney cancer datasets, aiming to identify potential therapeutic targets with high translational relevance. Using robust bioinformatics tools and datasets, the researchers identified several genes that were significantly overexpressed in RCC tumor tissues compared to normal kidney samples. These genes were selected based on thresholds of $\log_2$ fold change ($\log_2FC > 1$) and statistical significance ($p < 0.001$), ensuring that only the most promising candidates were considered. Expression validation was further confirmed using the TNMplot tool, which provided additional evidence for the upregulation of these genes in cancerous tissues.

To assess the potential therapeutic value of the identified targets, the study conducted prognostic analyses using Kaplan-Meier survival curves. The results showed that several of the identified targets were significantly associated with patient survival outcomes, with hazard ratios ($HR \neq 1$, $p < 0.05$) indicating their relevance as risk factors or protective markers in RCC progression. These findings suggest that these targets could have prognostic value and may be useful in guiding treatment decisions.

Druggability assessment of the identified targets was conducted using databases such as DGIdb, Open Targets, and DrugBank, which provided information on existing drugs with known interactions to the targets of interest. The study cross-verified these findings with existing literature to ensure that only pharmacologically actionable targets were retained for further investigation. To predict potential interactions with FDA-approved drugs, the researchers used the Drug Target Binding Affinity (DTBA) model. This model helped identify drugs with high binding affinity for the targets, which could be prioritized for further clinical evaluation. Notably, several of the drugs identified had established safety profiles in other malignancies, making them strong candidates for rapid repurposing in RCC treatment.

Tables 6.10 and 6.11 in the study provide detailed information on the identified kidney cancer targets, validated for their expression, prognostic significance, and druggability, as well as the top FDA-approved drugs predicted to have high binding affinity for these targets. This comprehensive approach offers a systematic framework for expanding the therapeutic options available for kidney cancer, particularly by focusing on repurposing existing drugs. The results have the potential to address some of the current limitations in RCC treatment and support the development of more personalized and effective therapeutic strategies tailored to individual patients with renal malignancies. This work exemplifies the power of integrating computational methods and experimental validation in the search for new cancer therapies, contributing to the growing field of precision oncology.

6.5 Conclusion

This work introduces a novel and integrated neuro-symbolic framework for identifying therapeutic targets and repurposing drugs in cancer, with a focus on enhancing precision oncology. By combining multi-omics data, deep learning models, and expert-driven symbolic rules, the study effectively addresses challenges related to drug-target prediction and the complexity of cancer biology. The approach not only identifies promising therapeutic targets but also provides actionable drug repurposing candidates, prioritizing FDA-approved drugs with established safety profiles for rapid translational application. Key findings demonstrate significant improvements in model performance, particularly in terms of interpretability and predictive accuracy, as evidenced by the neuro-symbolic fusion of symbolic logic and neural learning. The results underscore the value of this framework in expanding the therapeutic options available for cancers like kidney, breast, lung, and bladder, offering potential solutions to current treatment limitations. As cancer heterogeneity remains a significant obstacle in effective treatment, this research paves the way for personalized, data-driven therapeutic strategies. Future work will focus on further refining the models, incorporating additional biological data types, and validating predicted targets in clinical settings to foster real-world application and accelerate the path toward precision oncology.

CHAPTER 7

CONCLUSION AND FUTURE WORK

This doctoral research presents an integrated and multi-layered framework for computational drug discovery, uniting three complementary objectives drug-target interaction (DTI) prediction, drug-disease association (DDA) prediction, and explainable neuro-symbolic therapeutic target identification. The collective outcomes of these studies demonstrate a holistic approach to drug repurposing, addressing critical challenges in data imbalance, model interpretability, biological complexity, and translational applicability. Each component contributes uniquely to a comprehensive pipeline that bridges molecular data representation, graph-based learning, and interpretable neuro-symbolic reasoning for precision drug discovery.

The first objective, focused on Drug-Target Interaction and Binding Affinity Prediction, introduced two advanced deep learning models optimized for performance and robustness in imbalanced biochemical datasets. The 1D CNN-Self Attention-LSTM (SA-LSTM) hybrid model integrated with Honey Badger Optimization (HBO) successfully captured both local and sequential dependencies in drug and protein sequences. By incorporating a hierarchical embedding approach, clustering-based SMOTE oversampling, and adaptive hyperparameter tuning, this model effectively mitigated class imbalance and improved generalization. Experimental validation on benchmark datasets such as Davis and KIBA revealed substantial accuracy gains compared to baseline models, confirming the utility of hybrid architectures for molecular sequence understanding.

The second architecture, FusionNet, leveraged 1D CNNs, BiLSTMs, and Transformers optimized via the Layer-wise Adaptive Moments (LAMB) optimizer, achieving scalability and stable convergence even on large biochemical datasets. The inclusion of multi-head attention mechanisms enhanced the model's ability to learn long-range dependencies between drug and protein substructures, thereby improving binding affinity estimation. Together, these DTI frameworks established a robust foundation for downstream drug repurposing and target prioritization tasks by accurately modeling molecular interactions that underpin therapeutic potential.

www.ingramcontent.com/pod-product-compliance
Lightning Source LLC
LaVergne TN
LVHW010728061126
851857LV00014B/1384
* 9 7 8 1 9 6 2 1 1 6 4 2 8 *